BRIAN

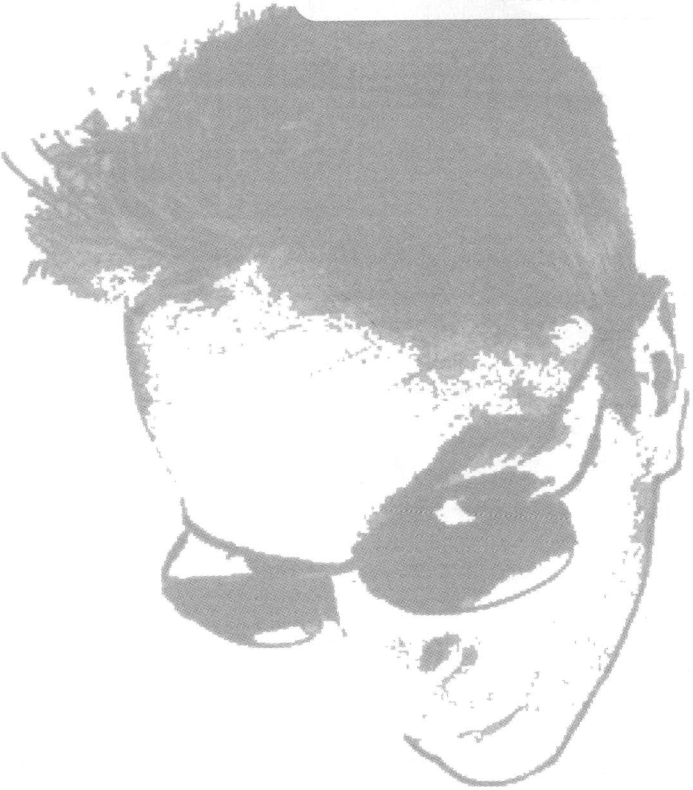

EYE-WIRED MEN

What Every Man Needs to Know About Himself

Discover the Keys to Being the Man that God Designed You to be, a God-Made Man

Unless otherwise indicated, all Scripture quotations are taken from the *King James Version* of the Bible.

The Scripture quotations marked AMP are taken from *The Amplified Bible, New Testament,* copyright © 1958, 1987 by The Lockman Foundation, La Habra, California; or from *The Amplified Bible, Old Testament,* copyright © 1964, 1987 by Zondervan Publishing House, Grand Rapids, Michigan.

The Scripture quotations marked NLT are taken from the *Holy Bible, New Living Translation,* copyright © 1996, 2004. Used by permission of Tyndale House Publishers, Inc., Carol Stream, Illinois 60188. All rights reserved.

The Scripture quotation marked NEB is take from the *New English Bible*, copyright © 1961, Oxford University Press, Oxford, England.

The Scripture quotation marked Deane Translation is from Deane, Anthony C., *St. Paul and His Letters*, Hodder and Stoughton, London, England, n.d.

EYE-WIRED MEN – *What Every Man Needs to Know About Himself*
ISBN # 1-893019-65-9

Brian Bohrer Ministries
P. O. Box 1577
Washington, Missouri 63090 U.S.A.
pastorbrian.org
636.239.5944

Cover Design: Jason Martin
Editor: Marilyn Price
Text Design: Lisa Simpson

24/7 Faith Publications
XXXFaith.com

What Others Have To Say About *Eye-Wired Men*

I have known Pastor Brian for 25 years and have personally seen him grow and mature into a great pastor and minister of the gospel of Jesus Christ. Pastor Brian's book, *Eye-Wired Men*, is a great tool that will help men get out and stay out of the trap the enemy has set to destroy their lives, their families, and really this generation. I would highly recommend this book to all men who want to live in the freedom and victory that Christ has purchased for us.

—Mark Hankins
Mark Hankins Ministries

God's Word says if you know the truth and you're willing to live it, the truth will make you free. Because this book is based on the Word of God, I believe it is anointed to destroy yokes and remove burdens from men who have been held in bondage by addictive behavior and spiritual strongholds. Pastor Brian has dealt with some tough subject matter and he didn't pull any punches. So read on, enjoy, and be free today, in Jesus' name.

—Dr. Mylon Le Fevre
Minister of the Gospel
Grammy and Dove Award Winner

When a man is drowning, he may grab at anything that resembles a rope. The problem is the rope may not be anchored or able to pull him to safety. The great thing about this book is it is anchored, giving the reader total reliance upon the promise of God through His Word.

Our hope comes from God and His hope never disappoints. The deception of pornography is the seemingly inescapable trap in which it snares men. The truth is God is the Deliverer and is always faithful to deliver us.

Brian Bohrer gives this truth in a relatable way for every man who reads this book.

—Bill Scheer
Pastor of Guts Church, Tulsa, Oklahoma

It is seldom that a writer decides to become transparent and deal with the deep-seated challenges facing our culture... This is one of those times... *Eye-Wired* is a Wide Open View of one of the greatest traps in Hell's arsenal facing our society... Brian is open... Sincere and willing to lay it on the line... As I read these pages I could not put it down and couldn't stop asking Heaven for a "Greater Purity." Every man in America needs to embrace the "Way of Escape" outlined on these pages... May Heaven Help us All... Thank you Brian for such a riveting book...

—Dr. Robert D. Thompson
Co-Chairman, The Gabriel Call
President, Intl. College of Excellence
President, Robb Thompson International
Chairman, Excellence in Ministry Intl.
Founder, Family Harvest

Contents

Introduction
The Red Lizard

C. S. Lewis wrote the book, *The Great Divorce,* to show the differences between heaven and hell. In this allegory, people take a day trip to the bright borders of heaven. Because heaven is so real, the people appear as ghosts next to the solidity of heaven and heaven's residents.

Here is a brief summary of a portion of Lewis's book that gives us an insightful allegory as to how lust consumes us and how difficult it is to deal radically with sexual sin. But it also shows us that once desire is conquered, it can become a great power to lead us onward in attaining the God-purpose for which we were created.

We'll look at one guest in heaven, whom we will call "Ghost," who carried a little red lizard on his shoulder. This lizard twitched and continually whispered things into Ghost's ears. At one point, Ghost snarled with impatience and told the lizard to shut up. Yet the red lizard continued to whisper into his ears.

In an encounter with a resident of heaven, an angel, Ghost explained that the lizard was insistent about coming with him to heaven, but he acknowledged that the red lizard's "stuff" simply wasn't acceptable for heaven. Therefore, he would have to leave and take the reptile home with him.

The angel offered to kill the red lizard, which would shut him up, but Ghost refused to allow such a drastic measure to be taken. Yet the angel insisted that it was the only way the lizard would ever shut up. Ghost explained that he just wanted it silenced, not killed.

The rhetoric continues back and forth between Ghost and the angel, with the angel insisting that the red lizard must be killed, as there was no other way to deal with him.

Suddenly, cognizant of the death threat upon its life, the lizard began making all kinds of promises to Ghost as to how nice he would be if he wouldn't let the angel kill him. Ghost felt that the burning power of the angel would kill him too. The angel told Ghost that it would be better to be dead than to live with this creature. Finally, Ghost relented and told the angel to do what he wanted. The angel gripped the lizard, then flung it onto the turf with its back broken.

Once Ghost saw what he thought was the end of red lizard, right before his eyes he saw the creation of an immense man, naked, not much smaller than the angel.

Then, shockingly, the lizard began struggling, and as it struggled, it grew and changed into a gigantic stallion – the greatest one Ghost had ever seen.

After embracing the feet of the angel, the newly made man leaped onto the horse's back, waved farewell to the angel, nudged the stallion, and they were off.

They vanished into the brilliance of heaven's morning light.[1]

The "red lizard" in the life of every man must be silenced – the whispers, lust, perversions, addictions, and temptations. Only then can the new man emerge, resulting in wholeness and intimacy in his marriage relationship. And only then can the man realize the God-given potential within him and develop it to the max.

With God there are no limitations or impossibilities. By discovering the truths in God's Lifestyle Manual – the Bible – you can become the God-made man He has called you to be!

Brian Bohrer

1

EVERY MAN'S ATTRACTION

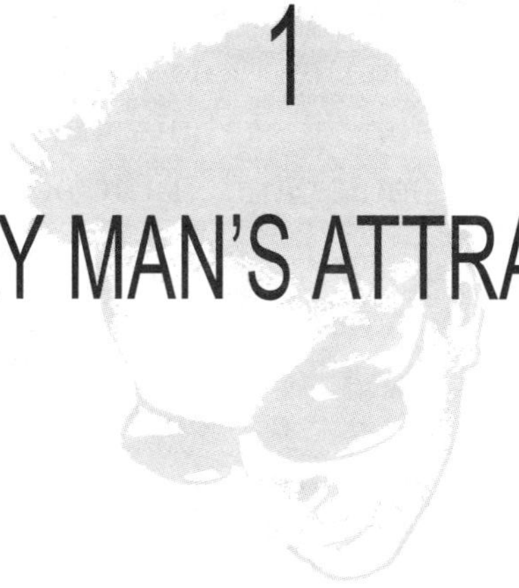

As I sat writing this book, my mind was debating whether I should quit or keep on going. The reason why I wanted to quit is because of the fear of rejection from the mainstream Christian community and my peers who would think I have lost my mind in putting together such a book as this.

During the time I worked on this project, it seemed that everything in my life that I believed in was tested, and at times I did not know if my whole world was going to come crashing down. It seemed that the enemy was trying to stop me from putting this project together and his very presence was eerie at times. Could it be that I struck a nerve in the core of his kingdom, or was this just a figment of my own imagination at work and just cycles of problems arising all at the same time? Who knows? Only eternity will tell what was going on.

At one of the biggest challenges during this time of writing, I decided to lay this project down because who was I to knock on the devil's door looking for trouble. I have always heard that you should not stir up more devils than you can cast out and it seemed that I had done just that. At one of my lowest points and at the point of giving up on what you are about to read, I turned on the TV to allow my mind to escape the pressure and to regain a sense of normalcy. I found my motivation to keep going in one of America's favorite people, Oprah!

I FOUND MY MOTIVATION TO KEEP GOING IN ONE OF AMERICA'S FAVORITE PEOPLE, OPRAH!

I must tell you the truth, I was not an Oprah fan nor did I have anything against her. I can honestly say that I have not watched her program more than four or five times in my life, but that day was the day that gave me the inspiration to keep going. That day as I sat watching Oprah she was interviewing Kirk Franklin, and boy, was I shocked in what he had to say about being addicted to pornography!

Kirk Franklin was and has always been my favorite singer and entertainer, and I am very proud of Kirk for his honesty and openness about an issue that lives in the darkness and he was bold enough to drag it into the light. His courage fed my courage to keep going and to speak boldly on the subject of manhood and what every man needs to know about himself.

As you will see, porn and lust have an effect on every man from the beginning of time to now because the Bible says, **"Every man is tempted."** The book you hold in your hands has the road map, God's GPS system, to lead you to a life of understanding and then to a life of freedom. I did not write this book intentionally to be a best seller but to be a lifesaver. Don't quit now. Keep on going and you will discover the keys to being the man that God designed you to be, a God-made man.

Every Man is Tempted

> **But every man is tempted, when he is drawn away of his own lust, and enticed.**
>
> **James 1:14**

Attraction – "That which catches our attention, catches our eye, catches our thoughts, and catches our mind."

To be equipped to become a man of God, you have to come out of denial into honesty. As you become older, you may think some things will just go away with time, but this scripture – our foundation scripture – says, **"Every man is tempted."**

There is a battle going on between the inward man and the flesh or carnal man. The carnal, fleshly man actually lives within the mind and we will call him the little red lizard from time to time. The carnal mind or the little red lizard controls the direction of his life until he is born again of the Spirit of God. (John 3:3.)

Yet I have seen people who are born again, who claim to be filled with the Holy Spirit, still live a life of bondage. Why? It is because many do not go through the process called "renewing the mind." Renewing the mind is the cleansing process from thoughts of lust that if they were told out loud, you would be totally embarrassed by them.

I like this statement that I heard a person say, "The mind does not stay renewed any more than your hair stays combed." Your mind will not be cleansed without renewing it to God's Word and it will not stay clean without daily meditating upon who you are in Christ. You have to continue to renew your mind to the Word of God if you are going to walk in victory over the thoughts of lust. The only thing which has power to kill the little red lizard is the power of the Word spoken by a new creation in Christ with a mind renewed to believe the Truth.

YOUR MIND WILL NOT BE CLEANSED WITHOUT RENEWING IT TO GOD'S WORD.

The Bible says, **"And be not conformed to this world: but be ye transformed by the renewing of your mind..."** (Romans 12:2). *The New Living Translation* says, **"Let God transform you into a new person by changing the way you think...."**

Maybe you have been controlled by lust (the little red lizard) and selfishness, but you can be a changed person. Let God transform you into a new person by changing the way you think. Take the thoughts of Jesus, and make them your own. Believe the Truth, and you will be made over again.

LET GOD TRANSFORM YOU INTO A NEW PERSON BY CHANGING THE WAY YOU THINK.

Men are driven by the way they think. The thought patterns then feed the imagination which directs your life. It is the revealed knowledge of the Word of God that will enable you to walk in freedom from unclean thoughts. Living under the influence of the Holy Spirit keeps your mind filled with holiness.

God will set an honest man free. If you become honest and drag things out of darkness into the light, you can be set free.

Let's read James 1:14 again: **"But every man is tempted, when he is drawn away of his own** (the little red lizard) **lust, and enticed."** We tend to blame a lot of things on the devil, but let's look at him through the eyes of the Scriptures.

We must remember that Satan is a spiritual being; he has no authority over us in the spiritual world. The only power that Satan has is the power that we give him by yielding to his thoughts. (See Ephesians 4:27.) The battle over who would control our spirits was fought by Christ, and Satan lost. So the battle for your spirit is over, once you accept Jesus Christ as your Savior. Satan's authority over you has been broken. (See Colossians 1:13-14.)

THE BATTLE THAT WE FACE TODAY IS WHO IS GOING TO RULE OUR MINDS, OUR THOUGHTS, AND OUR IMAGINATIONS.

The battle that we face today is who is going to rule our minds, our thoughts, and our imaginations. If we begin renewing our minds we are enabled to break free from lust, and with the weapon of God's Word we can destroy the little red lizard.

If you think you can live your life in this three-dimensional world without being tempted, you've got another think coming. You need to guard yourself, realizing that you will be tempted. The Bible tells you in this verse that you will be drawn away **"of your own lust,"** your own red lizard.

James 1:14 in *The Amplified Bible* says, **"But every person is tempted when he is drawn away, enticed and <u>baited by his own evil desire</u> (lust, passions)."** Baited by your own red lizard of lust and passions!

2

THE ENTICEMENT

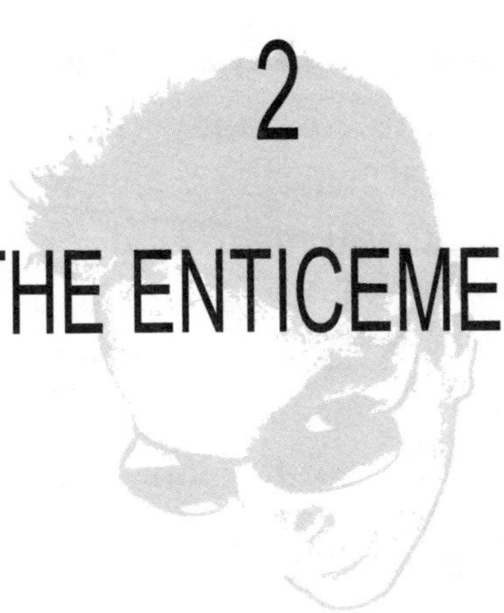

How many of you have ever been fishing? I spent a lot of money buying baits and trying to get the latest ones so I could catch more fish. When you fish with a lure, the lure will try to bait the fish to take the hook. One lure that I used to fish with was called a "rattletrap." It had something inside of it that made noise. A bass would be drawn to it by the noise and grab hold of that thing. This is what the enemy does with lust. He puts it out there where you can see it. He wants you to take it and be hooked with it.

Many times when you play with lust, once in a while you get away, but be it known unto you: *You won't always get away with it,* because one day the enemy (the red lizard) will sink in the hook. Then he will reel you in and put you in his boat. Eventually he's going to fillet you, mill you, and drop you in the grease. Then he will pull you out of the grease, put salt and pepper on you, dip you in some Louisiana hot sauce, and devour you. That's what lust does – that's what the red lizard does.

Lust is a deception, and the way you overcome it is by admitting that you are tempted with it. You may walk around in the Christian movement with a halo and say, "Pastor, you will never find me confessing that I have lust or anything about this red lizard living within me, because I believe in a positive confession." You have to look to the Scriptures and realize that there are things that will try to get into your life.

IN COMPARING PORNOGRAPHY TO A TATTOO, YOU RECEIVE A TATTOO ON YOUR ARM IN PAIN, BUT YOU WEAR IT IN PLEASURE. HOWEVER, PORNOGRAPHY IS JUST THE OPPOSITE. YOU RECEIVE IT IN PLEASURE, BUT THEN YOU WEAR IT IN PAIN.

The Adult Industry

The danger with pornography is that it works in the soul of man, bringing an image into the mind. In comparing pornography to a tattoo, you receive a tattoo on your arm in pain, but you wear it in pleasure. However, pornography is just the opposite. You receive it in pleasure, but then you wear it in pain.

Did you know that the adult industry in America (magazines, movies, and the Internet) generates over $13 billion a year and in the world the porn industry produces over $59 billion a year? That's more than Hollywood, Major League Baseball, the NBA, and the NFL combined. All of this adult pornography is feeding the red lizard within the mind of people and raising up a red lizard generation. The sad thing about it is that the more we see it on TV, the more we are desensitized by it; we are getting used to seeing things like "Girls Gone Wild," and Paris Hilton with hardly anything on. What was considered raunchy is now considered sexy. What is more shocking than that is the largest groups of people viewing Internet porn are kids between the ages of twelve and seventeen.

I was watching the Discovery channel and they were showing a story about grandmas who are sixty years of age, wanting to get their tattoos removed, because their grandchildren are looking at them. It's never wise to put a person's name on your arm, because tattoos usually outlast relationships. The program on the Discovery channel was showing grandmas going through the pain of tattoo removal through laser treatments.

> THERE IS ONLY ONE THING THAT HAS THE POWER TO REMOVE THE TATTOO OF LUST FROM THE SOUL OF MAN AND THAT IS THE ENGRAFTED WORD.

There is only one thing that has the power to remove the tattoo of lust from the soul of man and that is the engrafted Word, which is able to save your soul. (James 1:21.) It has the power, a process, and a mechanism within itself to get into your soul and remove the images that have been layered upon your imagination. The engrafting process has power to kill the red lizard of lust.

Recently I was ministering in a men's meeting. A man walked up to me after we closed and he said, "Pastor, I need some help." He said, "Lady Lust is a 'B*!#h' and she's got me by the 'b@!?s.'"

I talked to this gentleman and I shared a few things with him; mainly that if you're not sitting under the Word of God, it's hard to get help. Many times ministers have moved over into the realm of psychologists and therapists, but we cannot help someone just by counseling them. *It takes the power of the engrafted Word of God to set a man free, and it takes the Word of God to keep a man free.*

To stay free, you must submit to a mentorship program, submit to accountability, and allow your brain to be washed with the Word! John 15:3 says, **"Now ye are clean through the word which I have spoken unto you."** The Word of God has the power to cleanse your mind and your thoughts.

In Psalm 119:9-11 David said:

> **Wherewithal shall a young man cleanse his way? by taking heed thereto according to thy word.**
>
> **With my whole heart have I sought thee: O let me not wander from thy commandments.**
>
> **Thy word have I hid in mine heart, that I might not sin against thee.**

Jesus was tempted in the mind the same way you and I are tempted. We will be tempted in our thought life. The enemy always wants to take you further into deception until you lose your freedom. But God wants to give you a life of honor and power.

3

EYE-WIRED MEN

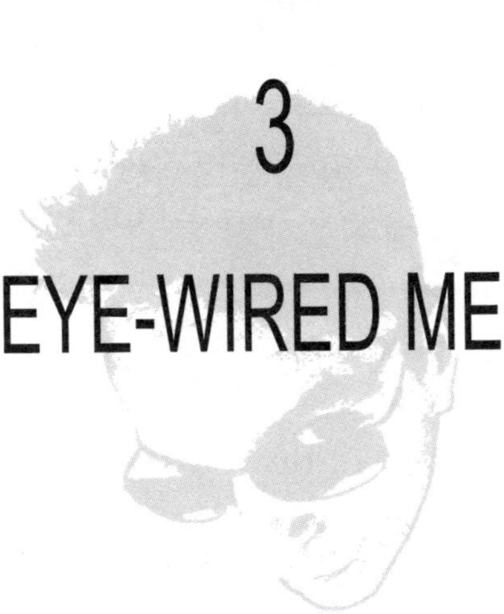

A man can undress a woman without undressing her, simply through his imagination. Actually, he can have sex with a woman without having sex with her physically because the imagination is so vivid. A man can fantasize with his mind because men are driven differently than women. Women are driven and stimulated by words of affection and by touch, while men are stimulated by their eyes and what they see in their imaginary world.

> MEN ARE EYE-DRIVEN AND EYE-WIRED. WHAT THEY SEE HAS AN EFFECT ON THEM.

Men are eye-driven and eye-wired. What they see has an effect on them. They like blondes, red Corvettes, black bras and panties, and anything that is sensual. The whole bra and panties industry is geared towards men to lure them and to feed the red lizard that lives within the mind of a man. That's why David said, **"I will set no wicked thing before mine eyes . . ."** (Psalm 101:3). You have to learn to starve your eyes, and if you want control of your life, you have to control and starve your thoughts. What goes in the eye gate has an effect upon your thoughts.

For you to be the God-made man, you have to have a pre-planned strategy to walk in victory. You can't just say, "Que sera sera, whatever will be will be. I'm just going to do my own thing making up life as I go." You have to stand guard. When you get up in the morning, make a decision to say what Job 31:1 *New Living Translation* says: **"I made a covenant with my eyes not to look with lust at a young woman."** What you look at today feeds the red lizard of lust within the mind and he will conquer you as long as you feed him.

Chemical Rush

Robb Weiss, the president of Sexual Recovery Institute, said on CNN (The Glenn Beck Show): "Internet pornography is the crack cocaine of sex addiction. And what we've been able to tell in the last few years is that, on MRIs, when you see a sex addict's brain light up around sexual stimulation, it looks like a cocaine addict."

WHEN LUST IS ENGAGED IN THE IMAGINATION, A CHEMICAL IS RELEASED INTO THE PLEASURE CENTER OF THE BRAIN.

When lust is engaged in the imagination, a chemical is released into the pleasure center of the brain. The pleasure center of the brain is where serotonin, dopamine, and endorphin levels are released into the mind. These chemicals are called the "feel good" chemicals that everyone is searching for. They control how we feel if we are happy or sad and high or low. It's the same high that people get from taking methamphetamines and other drugs. When a person is on methamphetamines the serotonin level in their brain is lifted to a higher level. This is called a chemical rush.

This chemical rush is the same rush that gamblers feel when they win the big one and these chemicals are released in the brain when people are thinking about winning at gambling, horse races, online betting, or watching porn. What people do not know is that this chemical rush is addictive and is part of the plan of the red lizard to dominate you and to control your life. According to Pure Life Ministries, 50 percent of all Christian men are addicted to porn. Porn is the fastest growing addiction among senior citizens.

What makes the difference between a God-made man and a perverted self-made man, or a man who is in the joint (prison) right now who has been caught as a predator? All predators were normal people at one time, but they yielded their thoughts and imagination to produce images that over time caused an action. A God-made man is a man, not just a male. We know you are a male because you have the goods; you were born with them. But to be a God-made man you will have to be born again and kill the red lizard and the desires of sexual addiction, money, power, porn, drugs, and everything else that is out of control.

4

THE ENEMY WITHIN

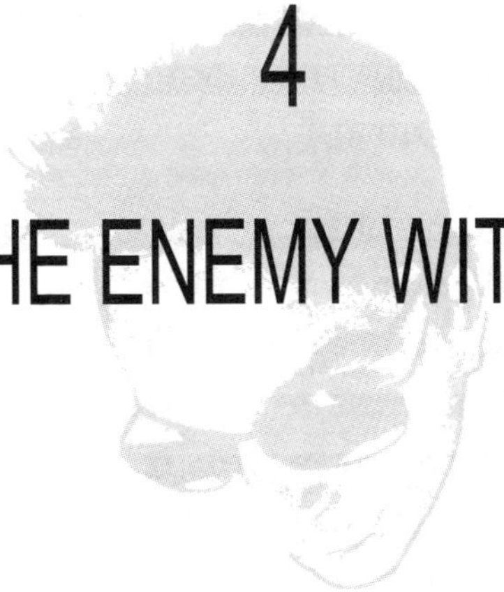

James 1:15 says, **"Then when lust hath conceived, it bringeth forth sin: and sin, when it is finished, bringeth forth death."**

There are several meanings for the word "lust":

- Excitement of the mind;
- Longing for what is forbidden;
- Passion, inordinate affection; and
- Coveting or setting your heart on something.

When it comes to lust, I am not only talking about lusting after a female. You can lust after money. The desire or greed for more has controlled many people. Lust, as well as the desire for power, fame, and fortune, can bring ruin to a man. The fact is that lust is not just a man thing. It is a woman thing also. It has been said that men crave to watch porn and women are satisfied to perform porn. Women feel important in the performance of porn; both are trapped in the red lizard industry. Not only are we concerned about the men who are trapped by the addiction of pornography, but we are equally concerned about the women who are trapped in the industry of pornography.

You must understand who your enemy is. The enemy is lust and it tries to control your mind. It's not the enemy on the outside that destroys you. It's the enemy within. He first showed up in the garden and this term **"said unto the woman"** is in Genesis, chapter 3, three times and the term **"Unto the woman he said"** is used one time. Lust is words and thoughts in the mind that are not in agreement with what God's Word is saying. We see the end result of what lust can do in Genesis 3:6: **"And when the woman saw that the tree was good for food, and that it was pleasant to the eyes, and a tree to be desired to make one wise, she took of the fruit thereof, and did eat, and gave also unto her husband with her; and he did eat."** This is the first beguiled man who walked on the face of the earth, and he produced many to follow. Most of you are one or you are married to one.

The Gates to the Soul

First John 2:16-17 says:

> **For all that is in the world, the lust of the flesh, and the lust of the eyes, and the pride of life, is not of the Father, but is of the world.**
>
> **And the world passeth away, and the lust thereof: but he that doeth the will of God abideth for ever.**

There are several gates to the soul, but the main gate is the eye gate. That's why the enemy plots through the media today to get into the soul of man. Everything that you see on television is not only designed to entertain you, but it is designed to deceive you. The devil cannot defeat you unless he first deceives you. That is why when you drive down the interstate and see sexually explicit advertisements, it draws in the man's eyes. It's like a magnet.

THERE ARE SEVERAL GATES TO THE SOUL, BUT THE MAIN GATE IS THE EYE GATE. THAT'S WHY THE ENEMY PLOTS THROUGH THE MEDIA TODAY TO GET INTO THE SOUL OF MAN.

There is such an exposure to hard core pornography on the Internet today that the enemy targets ministers and godly men among those he desires to bring down. When an image is in the mind long enough, it will create an action and form a lifestyle.

Lance Tracy, a recovering porn addict, led a study on the effects of porn. Tracy exposed men to pornography over a thirty-day period in which he found that these men were increasingly stimulated everywhere they went by all the women they saw and less and less stimulated by their partners.

This is the hard proof that porn destroys marriages and it destroys the honor of being a man. You know that you are swimming with the sharks when you are going behind your wife's back to buy pornography and

> YOU KNOW THAT YOU ARE SWIMMING WITH THE SHARKS WHEN YOU ARE GOING BEHIND YOUR WIFE'S BACK TO BUY PORNOGRAPHY AND WHEN YOU ARE WATCHING PORN ON THE INTERNET IN THE MIDDLE OF THE NIGHT WHILE SHE IS SLEEPING.

when you are watching porn on the Internet in the middle of the night while she is sleeping.

Soon the secret will be out. You will feel the pain when she discovers the hidden secret of your life. Many marriages have been destroyed because of the red lizard that is fed so well within the hidden soul of a man. Just think how you are going to feel the day you get caught with one hand on your mouse and the other hand in your own pants. It is time now to be clean and to be free.

5

THE MIND HAS PROCREATIVE POWER

The mind has procreative power. First Peter 1:13 says, **"Gird up the loins of your mind...."** The loins of a man are his genitals – the part of man involved in intercourse, and through intercourse the woman conceives. You must guard the loins of your mind.

> YOU HAVE TO GIRD UP THE LOINS OF YOUR MIND, BECAUSE YOUR MIND CAN REPRODUCE WHAT IS SEEN THROUGH THE EYE GATE.

Something in the mind can conceive and actualize into this three-dimensional world, because over a period of time it demands an action. As a man thinks in his heart, so is he. (See Proverbs 23:7.) He becomes what he thinks on. The eyes are never satisfied just looking. In time what is planted will grow a harvest and you will eat the fruit of it. (Proverbs 27:20.)

Your only answer to freedom is to regain your honor by honesty. Let God transform you into a new man by changing the way you think.

You have to gird up the loins of your mind, because your mind can reproduce what is seen through the eye gate. This is why men have trouble with masturbation. [From this point on, we will call masturbation the "Big M."] When you watch porn you begin to fantasize and then it leads to the "Big M." I'm not just talking about single men; married men have trouble with the Big M. Once again, the Big M is not just a male thing; it is a women thing also. According to Pure Life Ministries, 20 percent of Christian women struggle with porn.

Males who are exposed to pornography before the age of thirteen have a greater challenge sexually in life because a seed of perversion is planted within their minds. This should be a wake-up call to all people who are reading this book to watch out for your children and make sure that you do your best to keep trouble out of their minds.

Robert W. Peters, President of Morality in Media, quoted Naomi Wolf of *New York* magazine, saying that in Manhattan, more young women are discovering that a growing number of guys would rather stay home and look at pornography on the Internet – and, of course, masturbate to it – than have an actual real-life relationship with a woman.

Beware of Pornography

Perversion and iniquity are planted in the mind in several ways. You may have been abused sexually as a child; God will restore you. You could have been exposed to pornography as a child; God can heal you of that also. Perversion is planted when a person yields to twisted thinking by watching it; thus the human will becomes weak, the seed of iniquity gets planted within our minds. The result is guilt, which reproduces a cycle of shame. As we attempt to cover sin rather than confess it, it produces a type of rejection and a guilt-controlled personality.

PERVERSION IS PLANTED WHEN A PERSON YIELDS TO TWISTED THINKING BY WATCHING IT; THUS THE HUMAN WILL BECOMES WEAK.

In the next few chapters, we will show you the plan for freedom and how you can destroy Lady Lust.

6

MASTERING YOUR THOUGHTS

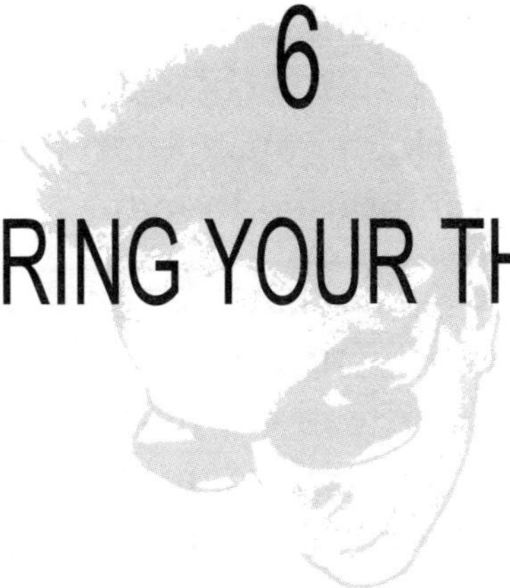

The Bible says, **"Let this mind be in you, which was also in Christ Jesus"** (Philippians 2:5). Jesus made His thoughts His servants. Similarly, you must make your thoughts your servants. If you don't, your thoughts will master you all of your life.

You can be filled with the Holy Spirit and still allow lustful thoughts to master you. Jesus mastered His thoughts. Not only was He a prototype of a man, He was a man. The Bible says He stripped Himself of His divine powers and became as a man. (Philippians 2:7-8.)

Hebrews 4:15 says, "[He] **was in all points tempted like as we are, yet without sin."**

We know that Jesus was tempted in Luke, chapter 4, and in Matthew, chapter 4. He was tempted the same way you and I are tempted. When the devil came to Jesus in the wilderness, he did not appear in the

THE BATTLEGROUND IS YOUR MIND AND YOUR THOUGHTS. THAT'S WHERE THE DEVIL WILL TEMPT YOU.

three-dimensional world wearing a red suit, hoofs, horns, and a pitchfork, because that is not an equal temptation to man.

The battleground is your mind and your thoughts. That's where the devil will tempt you. What is in your mind will happen in time because the mind has the ability to procreate an action. It has magnetism. It can draw in iniquity. If uncontrolled, it will force a man to get out of his bed at 11:00 at night, go downtown, pay $75 to get a BJ and visit a prostitute.

The Bible warns us in the book of Proverbs about the strange woman, Lady Lust, who has power to lure you in and eventually take your soul and your honor. (See Proverbs 2:16; 5:3; 5:20; 6:24; 7:5; 20:16; 23:27; 27:13.) Proverbs also tells you about another woman called Lady Wisdom who is able to cause you to be a man of honor and a man in control of your emotions. Remember, Lady Lust is not a lady; she is a master who takes away your freedom.

LUST IS THE STRANGE WOMAN WHO LIVES IN THE MIND. BUT YOU DO HAVE POWER OVER YOUR THOUGHTS.

Who is this woman? This woman, "Lady Lust – the red lizard," is the strange woman whom Solomon warns you about. Lust is the strange woman who lives in the mind. You see a woman walking into church or a co-worker, she smiles – one day she speaks. Though you are in covenant with a holy God, you open your heart to her, she listens. Or she plays on your manhood and needs you to care for her. You feel that she respects your opinion, values you. You begin to compare her to your wife. Know this, the strange woman is only looking to meet her own unmet needs. She is carnal rather than spiritual. Once you lose your family and your honor, she will find another life to destroy.

A Different Society

We live in a different society today than it was back in the day and things are becoming looser. Tops are lower, cleavage is in, revealing the belly and belly button rings are in, and so are tattoos on the lower back, and thongs (the whale's tail) are in plain sight.

As men we ought to say, "How dare women come around us bringing temptation like this to us? They shouldn't dress like that in the church."

You are right, but guess what? You are not always going to be in the church. It's not your eyes and your mind that are in the church that will defeat you. It is when you are alone in the mall or when you are driving down the road and you see a scantily dressed jogger. You'll drive five blocks to go back so you can get the right behind view!

What causes a person to drive around the block to take a second look? It is the red lizard that lives within. As I said before, the red lizard is lust, the strange woman who must be mastered and destroyed by God's

Word. As you meditate upon God's Word and take control of your mind by casting down imaginations and become the master of EVERY THOUGHT (2 Corinthians 10:5), you are on the road to freedom.

You do have power over your thoughts. What you see and hear feeds your thoughts and what you feed on will dominate you. When you feed on the things of God, they will dominate your thoughts, and your thoughts will become your lifestyle.

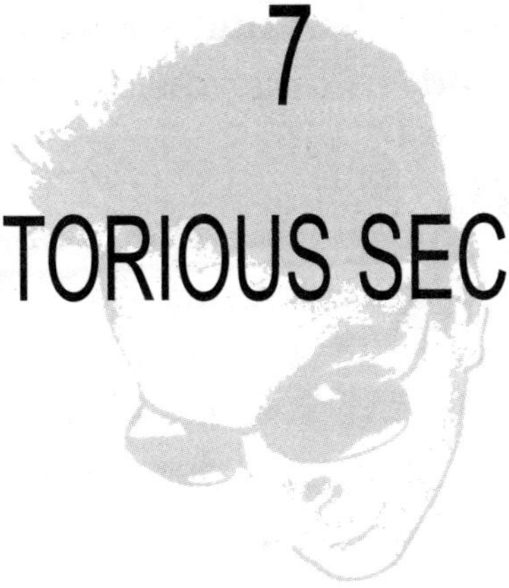

7

VICTORIOUS SECRETS

As men, we no longer have to be controlled by the *panty and bra catalogues* which are mailed to our homes. We can be controlled by ***victorious secrets!*** If any trashy magazines come to your house, get rid of them immediately or they will end up in your sons' hands.

Another area where you have to guard what you see is on the Internet. Men, and especially men in ministry, are targets of pornography on the Internet. The motive is to send porn to you on your personal computer.

There is a war going on, and there are five ways you can win this war over lust.

Ephesians 5:3 says, **"But fornication, and all uncleanness, or covetousness, let it not be once named among you...."** *The Amplified Bible* says, **"But immorality (sexual vice) and all impurity [of**

lustful, rich, wasteful living] or greediness must not even be named among you...."

"Fornication" is a sexual act between people who are not married. It is immorality. When Paul talked about "uncleanness," he was talking about impurity. The word "uncleanness" is not talking about your lack of physical hygiene. It is talking about bestiality and erotic, kinky, raw things that are taking place in the world.

TO BE A SUCCESSFUL GOD-MADE MAN, YOU WILL HAVE TO CONTROL TWO AREAS OF YOUR LIFE: ONE IS YOUR LOVE FOR MONEY AND THE OTHER IS YOUR CRAVING FOR SEX.

"Covetousness" is another type of lust. There is the love and lust for money and the love and lust to be rich. It's something that has to be controlled. To be a successful God-made man, you will have to control two areas of your life: One is your love for money and the other is your craving for sex. These are the two biggest things that men are faced with and they are strong desires today – sexual desires and the desire to be rich.

Paul says, **"But fornication, and all uncleanness, or covetousness, <u>let it not be once named among you</u>, as becometh saints."** Paul is saying that these issues – fornication, adultery, cheating, or any type of raw sexual act – should not even be named among us.

We have a mark that we need to strive for. All types of lust and things that are not clean have been named among us. We need those things removed. The Word of God has the principles that show us how to remove them.

You need to be honest about the issues that are driving you to do something you know you will regret later. You need to allow the Holy Spirit to control these issues before they turn you into a monster.

Some women are satisfied if they have sex once or twice a month because of their busy lifestyle and some women desire to have sex two or three times a week. However, the normal man desires sex three to five times a week. As a result, some wives think, *"I married a pervert."*

AS A HUSBAND YOU NEED TO LEARN HOW TO OPEN UP THE HEART OF YOUR WIFE, BECAUSE SHE DOESN'T WANT TO FEEL LIKE SHE IS A PROSTITUTE.

As a husband, you need to learn how to open up the heart of your wife, because she doesn't want to feel like she is a prostitute, just used for sexual pleasures. Sometimes the husband treats the wife bad all day long, but when it's 9:30 or 10:00 at night, the husband turns into Mr. Casanova again! That doesn't turn the wife on!

Sexual Purity

Men, you can win in this arena of sexual purity by building an arsenal within your life. This arsenal is made up of five things: accountability, mentoring, meditating on God's Word, managing your time, and integrity.

1. Accountability

You will never overcome lust without accountability. We are responsible for giving an account of our actions. There has not been a lot taught about accountability, which means men being submitted to other men, being answerable for your time and actions. Now, this doesn't mean that the man you are accountable to is a perfect man or that he has never had any problems. Those who have admitted and overcome are the best mentors.

YOU WILL NEVER BE ABLE TO HAVE ACCOUNTABILITY WITH ANYONE YOU DISCUSS YOUR SEX LIFE WITH IN A WRONG WAY.

You can find reliable, trustworthy men your own age or older, and be held accountable – requiring a person to take charge of, or be trusted with, important matters. But see that you do not betray this trust. The way you destroy it is by getting together and talking about your wives and your sex life:

- "Did you get any last night?"
- "No, my old lady wouldn't give me any."
- "Man, we really got some good stuff last night."

When men talk this way, they break down their intimacy level by sharing personal things about their wife with other men. You will never be able to have accountability with anyone you discuss your sex life with in a wrong way. It's not the will of God to discuss your sexual relationship with your wife with any other man unless it's an elder or someone who is going to help you overcome – someone you can go to with honesty and admit that you have a problem. An elder can pray with you and share with you how to touch your wife's heart and how to minister to her.

When you destroy accountability, you open the door to the devil. This is not a problem just with men. Women talk about sex and they like to have what we call "pillow talk." They like to talk about the situations that they are having with men and it's wrong. It's not scriptural. Women need to understand that they are destroying their husband when they discuss the performance or the lack of it with any other woman.

With nearly thirty years in ministry, women have told me every possible thing regarding their sex lives. You turn red and you are supposed to look at them and say, "Okay." Their situations are very real.

Now in my forties and as a man understanding more about the mind of a man, a lot of problems that women discuss with my wife and me are because there is no time for foreplay. There is selfishness rather than selflessness. When a man desires to get his own needs met alone and his wife does not respond, but withholds from him, a man gets angry. A man then feels rejected which causes anger, frustration, and sometimes it causes him to masturbate. Both husband and wife need to learn the sexual needs of each other and yield to the love of God rather than their selfish, self-centered desires. The desire to treat our husbands/wives the way the Bible tells us to comes from our desire to please God rather than ourselves. As a godly man you can no longer feed wrong desires and expect to perform well in the act of marriage with your wife and develop intimacy with her.

Accountability is very important to men. This means never discussing the act of marriage or sexual acts with any other male if it's not in a wholesome, correct way and if your accountability partner is not there to help you.

Our vision is to build a championship team of men – a winning team. Whatever it takes to win, we are going to do it. We are going to overcome. We are going to face these problems rather than live in denial. If you live in denial, you will never get help. You must be honest.

2. Mentoring

Another part of your arsenal is mentoring (tutoring and training). The biblical term for "mentoring" is discipleship. We don't see a lot of discipleship going on in the Body of Christ, but I heard the Lord say, "We want to get back to discipleship and disciple some men." I can't disciple everyone by myself. I don't have the time to disciple one-on-one like I did twenty years ago, but I can disciple a group of men who are willing to be discipled. Then they can turn around and disciple another. That's multilevel mentoring!

IF YOU WANT TO WIN, YOU HAVE TO BE OPEN TO BE MENTORED AND DISCIPLED.

If you want to win, you have to be open to be mentored and discipled. The word "disciple" in the Greek is *mathetes,* which means working through the problems and finding solutions. It's where we get the word "mathematics." There are problems in our lives and we have to work through these problems and find solutions.

3. Meditating

The third part of your arsenal is to meditate on God's Word. What you meditate on is what you will become. If you are meditating on wrong things in your imagination and in your mind, you are going to have the desire to have it performed in your life.

Proverbs 23:7 says, **"For as he thinketh in his heart, so is he. . . ."** Whatever you are thinking on, you will become. The meditation of your mind has to be on the things of God. The Bible talks about how to be free. It talks about different things that we are facing, but we have to control our meditation.

What you have to do is not just thought displacement. You have to do forced meditation. You have to be strong enough and have the desire, "I'm going to do something about my life, and the only way I'm going to do something about my life is change my thinking. My thinking is not going to change without a battle."

FANTASIZING DESTROYS THE MARRIAGE AND THE BOND OF INTIMACY.

Your thinking has more to do with your thoughts and your imagination. Imagination leads to fantasizing. Men fantasize and they fantasize with other people's wives and young girls. Fantasizing destroys the marriage and the bond of intimacy.

The "Big M" is a fantasy. Your thoughts and imaginations are connected with being aroused. If you want to change, you are going to have to force yourself to feed upon some scriptures that bring purity and a cleansing to your soul. A cleansing process has to take place. You have to have holiness branded on the inside of you.

Once a tattoo is on your skin, it's there to stay unless it is later removed through laser treatments. This is what happens in the realm of the soul. Lust is tattooed to your soul and you think, *I can quit anytime.* But when you try to quit, you are going to find out that it is embedded. You have to have supernatural power to have that thing removed from your life, because your soul has been tattooed. Your soul has been marred by lust. Your soul has been controlled by pictures and images that you have allowed to come to your eyes and to your senses. You have to control your meditation.

> GOD'S WORD WILL RELEASE HIS POWER AND PURITY INTO YOUR LIFE.

You ask, "What do I do?" You begin by meditating on the Word of God. Find scriptures about the authority of the believer and about purity and holiness and take time to meditate upon them by putting them on index cards and speak them to yourself every day. God's Word will release His power and purity into your life. He has given you the Holy Spirit; remember His first name, Holy. He is the abiding presence in you, teaching you, empowering you.

All of us need to move up a level in the areas of purity and holiness, whether it's in our thoughts, words, what we're watching, or what we are hearing, including the music we listen to which has an influence. Music is a powerful tool today – for good or for evil, depending on the kind you are listening to.

4. Managing Your Time

The fourth thing to add to your arsenal is learn to manage your time – what you are doing with your time and where you are spending your time. This, of course, falls under the category of accountability.

If you truly want to be free, you have to give an account of your time. Some men disappear and they go off into the city where they have X-rated theaters that show X-rated pornography. I'm talking about X-rated movies – hard-core pornography as well as movies about homosexuality and all types of things. As well as R-rated movies, they are rated for a reason. If you want to be free, you have to manage your time and give an account of your time.

IF YOU WANT TO BE FREE, YOU HAVE TO MANAGE YOUR TIME AND GIVE AN ACCOUNT OF YOUR TIME.

What are you doing when you are staying up late at night and your wife and children are asleep? What are you watching on television, or what have you got under the bed? Where did you get those videos? You go down to the rental place and go into the backroom. You have to make a choice that you are not going to the backroom. In fact, the backroom ought to be shut down. It's really a disgrace that we allow it to be open. As I said previously, we are fighting a spiritual battle.

What are you doing when you are on the Internet? If that becomes a problem, take drastic measures. I believe in drastic measures. The Bible believes in drastic measures. The Bible says, **"If your hand or your foot causes you to stumble and sin, cut it off and throw it away from you.... And if your eye causes you to stumble and sin, pluck it out and throw it away from you ..."** (Matthew 18:8-9 AMP). In other words, ask God to help you get control over the members of your body that are leading you into a carnal lifestyle rather than into a spiritual lifestyle.

YOU ARE NOT GOING TO BE FREE WITHOUT PAIN.

You are not going to be free without pain. If the Internet is controlling your life, try a filter, although you will still know ways to get around the filter. If you don't know how to inactivate the filter, your children will know how to unplug it. But if that thing is bothering you, you need to have accountability with someone and say, "Man, I'm watching things on the Internet that I know I shouldn't be watching. What do you think I need to do?" You need to unplug the Internet!

You need to ask yourself some serious questions, such as:

- Do you really want to be free?
- Do you want to be a pervert?
- Do you want to be bound?
- Do you want to destroy the intimacy that you have with God? With your wife?

- Do you want your children to know?
- How are you going to feel as a father when your kids find out that you have been watching R-rated movies, or is it X-rated now? And you think you're hiding this lifestyle?

It is best to get free right now and make it your testimony, because you're not going to be able to hide it. The devil is trying to set you up so he can expose you, and eventually he will expose you. If there are things hidden in your life and you think you can hide them, they will be exposed, so it's best to take drastic measures now.

5. Integrity

The fifth part of your arsenal to fight against lust is integrity. This means being truthful, honest, up-front, and faithful. Integrity is the missing ingredient to wholeness, so it has to come back into your life. It has to be your desire to be a man of integrity.

IT HAS TO BE YOUR DESIRE TO BE A MAN OF INTEGRITY.

When I was in my twenties, I found what I call a "theme scripture" when I realized that there was a battle going on in me for purity. There was a battle going on in my life, even though I was married and in the ministry. I wanted to be free, because I didn't want my past to control my future.

I began to meditate on Psalm 119:9: **"Wherewithal shall a young man cleanse his way? by taking heed thereto according to thy word."** *The*

Amplified Version says, **"By taking heed and keeping watch [on himself] according to Your word [conforming his life to it]."**

You can watch yourself by obeying God's Word. However, you can't watch yourself by yourself, because I don't want you to fail morally. I care about your children and your marriage enough that I do not want you to fail morally.

There is always an excuse for you to fail morally. There is an excuse to get caught up at the workplace. You meet someone on the job and she smells good and looks good. Your wife is not looking too good anymore. Your wife is complaining and putting on a little weight. But on the job you see Miss Priss. I'm here to tell you, Miss Priss is not what you think she is. She is what the Bible warns you about. She is a "strange woman," a flattering woman.

I have had many opportunities in every church I have pastored to fail morally. I've had women pinch me on the butt. I've had women make advances at me. I've had women wink at me. Greet me with a front hug, or sit in church across the aisle with a slit up to Dallas. I've had women write notes. I've had them give me their phone number. I want to tell you, 99 percent of the women who do this are married women. I realized that I have to stand guard and keep people around me, because I don't want to fall into a trap that has been laid.

David warned Solomon about the strange women who flatter you, woo you, and make sexual advances to you. Some men can't wait until a woman gives them a sexual advance. If it wasn't for the grace of God, they would have already failed morally. I'm talking about Christians who go to church every week.

"CAN A MAN TAKE FIRE IN HIS BOSOM, AND HIS CLOTHES NOT BE BURNED?" PROVERBS 6:27

I want to tell you the down side to it. It will cost you more than you are willing to pay. David told his son, **"Can a man take fire in his bosom, and his clothes not be burned?"** (Proverbs 6:27). He said, "What you are getting ready to do is to set a fire off on the inside of you. A world of iniquity is getting ready to start burning." You are going to have a hard time putting it out without the power of the Spirit of God.

How do you cleanse your ways? Basically, you cleanse your ways by taking heed to the Word. David said, **"With my whole heart have I sought thee: O let me not wander from thy commandments. Thy word have I hid in mine heart, that I might not sin against thee"** (Psalm 119:10-11). He said, "It's the Word that I have hidden in my heart that keeps me from sinning."

David missed the mark. In Psalm 51 he repents for missing the mark. He said, "I am willing to repent. My sin is open before everyone."

Proverbs 28:13 says, **"He that covereth his sins shall not prosper: but whoso confesseth and for-**

saketh them shall have mercy." David was saying, "I am not here to cover my sin. I am here to repent of my sin. I am here to get honest. I made a mistake. I failed morally." But he said, "I still want to be God's man. Whether the people follow me or not, I'm going to repent." Then he said:

> **Create in me a clean heart, O God; and renew a right spirit within me.**
>
> **Cast me not away from thy presence; and take not thy holy spirit from me.**
>
> **Psalm 51:10-11**

David was broken before Almighty God. Through his brokenness he became great, and through humility we become great.

A Word from Dr. Lester Sumrall

Years ago, the late Dr. Lester Sumrall, one of my heroes, came to preach in our church. Anyone named Lester is a friend of mine because my middle name is Lester. At this time, I was twenty-five years old, and he spoke into my life.

After the meetings at our church, I was to drive him back to the airport so he could fly out. When I went to his room to pick him up, I was shaking in my boots, because here is an old general who has been all over the world preaching the gospel and casting out devils. There was no way that he could look at you without seeing what's on the inside of you, so I was all proper when I went into his room.

He said, "Have a seat." So I sat down. He said, "I watched CNN news (before there was Fox News) so I would know what's going on in the world." Then he said, "There is no sense in lying about it." He went on to say that "God's greatest man David, God's strongest man Samson, and God's wisest man Solomon all fell because of lust."

Then he asked me, "You got a car?" I said, "Yes." He said, "Let's go for a ride." So he walked out and his two pilots and a multimillion-dollar jet were waiting on him.

We rode around and he said to me, "The only thing I can tell you is that you need to slay your giants while you are young or they will defeat you when you get old."

YOU NEED TO SLAY YOUR GIANTS WHILE YOU ARE YOUNG OR THEY WILL DEFEAT YOU WHEN YOU GET OLD.

He said, "There are several giants. One giant is lust for sex and you have to kill it. Another giant is the lust for money and you have to kill it. Another giant is the lust for power and you have to kill it. Those are the three evils – power, money, and sex." He said, "Every man has these three things on the inside of him. There is no sense in lying about it."

I was holding on to the steering wheel, and my handprint was embedded into it while Dr. Sumrall was talking to me!

Now, we have to kill our giants. We can't kill our giants by denying their power over us. There are giants in the land. Destroy your giants! The ***victorious secrets*** I am sharing with you will help you overcome and master those giants so you can be what God wants you to be and fulfill your destiny!

8

BREAKING FREE

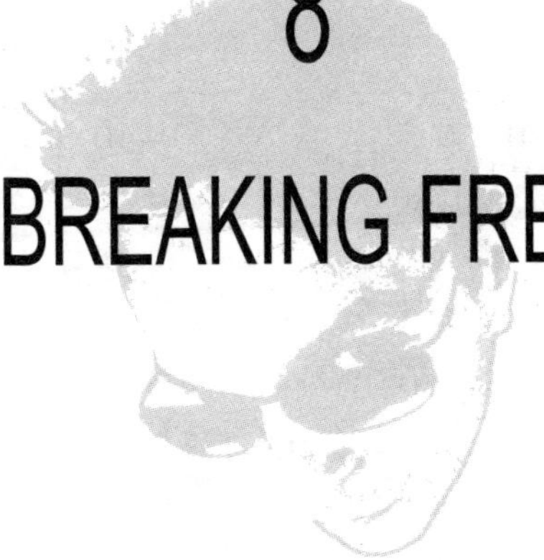

I write unto you, little children, because your sins are forgiven you for his name's sake.

I write unto you, fathers, because ye have known him that is from the beginning. I write unto you, young men, because ye have overcome the wicked one. I write unto you, little children, because ye have known the Father.

I have written unto you, fathers, because ye have known him that is from the beginning. I have written unto you, young men, because ye are strong, and the word of God abideth in you, and ye have overcome the wicked one.

1 John 2:12-14

Verse 14 lists our goal: <u>to overcome the wicked one</u>. John hits all ages of people: little children, fathers, and young men. He says of the young men, **"Ye are strong."** Why? **"The word of God abideth in you."**

Notice, John uses the word "abideth" rather than "abides." "Abideth" means it ever lives. It's a continuation of the word "abiding," not a one-time hearing the Word. It's not one time of getting into the Word. It's not one time going over a scripture. This word "abideth" means ever living, always continuing to live on the inside of you. John said, "This is the reason you are strong. No other reason. This is the reason you have overcome the wicked one."

LUST IS EVERY MAN'S BATTLE. WE WANT TO LEARN TO OVERCOME LUST AND NOT FEED IT, BUT LIVE AS MEN OF INTEGRITY.

"The wicked one" is not just the devil. The evil one we are looking at right now is lust and the powers that try to control and dominate men. Lust is every man's battle. We want to learn to overcome lust and not feed it, but live as men of integrity.

In verses 15-17, the apostle gives us some keys for overcoming:

> **Love not the world, neither the things that are in the world. If any man love the world, the love of the Father is not in him.**
>
> **For all that is in the world, the lust of the flesh, and the lust of the eyes, and the pride of life, is not of the Father, but is of the world.** [That's what we are dealing with right now.]

And the world passeth away, and the lust thereof: but he that doeth the will of God abideth for ever.

Now let's look at First John 3:3: **"And every man that hath this hope in him purifieth himself, even as he is pure."** The Apostle John is saying, "If you have this hope, you are going to purify yourself." This means there is a part you must play to be cleansed from lust, from the past, from greed, and from strongholds that keep men in bondage.

Men especially have a problem with lust, and we live in a world that feeds lust. Most men think, "*When I get married, I'll never have that problem again in my life. I can't wait to get married and I'll never have the problem with the 'Big M.'*"

It has been proven that 60 percent of men who are married masturbate because of frustration with a relationship, frustration with their wife, pressures on the job, and pressures to make money. Just because a person is married does not mean that they have conquered the lust problem. What we want to do is learn to conquer the lust problem by what I call ***victorious secrets.***

IT HAS BEEN PROVEN THAT THE MAJORITY OF ALL PORNOGRAPHY ENDS UP IN THE HANDS OF MINORS.

It has been proven that the majority of all pornography ends up in the hands of minors. A lot of people are exposed to pornography at a young age and that pornography begins to form iniquity. By "iniquity" I mean a path of destruction.

If the iniquity is greed, it produces a path of destruction. It causes a man to rob, steal, and cheat to do anything he possibly can to get money. But when it comes to pornography, the road of destruction is formed. It's not long that a young man has to feed that lust monster on the inside of him.

Psychologically, we find that the term for lust is "addictive behaviors." In Romans, chapter 7, Paul talks about a battle that is going on. I really believe that Paul is talking about the man under the law, how the man under the law cannot please God period. But Paul also mentions things that sound familiar to a lot of people.

In Romans 7:15 Paul says, **"For that which I do I allow not: for what I would, that do I not; but what I hate, that do I."** That's a lot of what I do and what I should do! But he said, "The things that I'm doing, I don't want to do." In other words, "I really hate what I'm doing, but I can't stop doing what I'm doing."

In verses 23-24 he says:

> **But I see another law in my members, warring against the law of my mind, and bringing me into captivity to the law of sin which is in my members.**
>
> **O wretched man that I am! who shall deliver me from the body of this death?**

Now, notice what Paul says in chapter 8, verses 1 and 2:

There is therefore now no condemnation to them which are in Christ Jesus, who walk not after the flesh, but after the Spirit.

For the law of the Spirit of life in Christ Jesus hath made me free from the law of sin and death.

Paul said, "There is a law that seems to be working in my members. I don't understand my actions." One translation says, "They [my actions] baffle or bewilder me." He said, "But the things I am practicing, I hate. I just don't know how to win over those things."

We read Ephesians 5:3 before, but let's read it again: **"But fornication, and all uncleanness, or covetousness, let it not be once named among you, as becometh saints** [or becometh men]**."** Paul was saying, "Let not fornication be named once among you." That's our goal, that fornication, uncleanness, or covetousness not be named one time among us as men.

The only way we can do that is by working together as men. Many men are isolated, and they have a lot of pressure on them today. That's why some run from the pressures and responsibilities that are placed upon them. As men we need each other. Each of us needs to find a friend who will help us be accountable, do what God has called us to do, and be what God wants us to be so we will not have fornication, uncleanness, or covetousness named among us one time.

We need to be transparent. Like an alcoholic who is addicted needs a support system, we as men need a support system and a sponsor where we can learn to sponsor and support someone else.

If I understand it right, when you enter A.A., someone has to sponsor you. I have a poker chip at home and it was my dad's. It's a certain color and that meant he had been sober for a certain number of months. Then, a year or so later, he would get another poker chip with a different color with a saying on it. You keep going year after year, but there comes a point where you can learn to sponsor someone else.

One man who had fifteen years of sobriety told me, "I have to guard myself from one drink. I can't allow any of that into my life, because I'll go right back to being an alcoholic."

There are addictive behaviors. Sexual addiction is one of them. If we don't learn how to gain control, one look will lead to a gaze and the next thing we know, we are back in the magazines, on the Internet, and renting videos. We are destroying our own soul, and the monster is alive on the inside of us. We look good on the outside, but there is something on the inside that is destroying us and feeding the wrong desires.

> SEXUAL ADDICTION IS JUST AS REAL AS DRUG ADDICTION, AND THE BATTLE BEGINS IN THE MIND.

Paul is saying, "I want to explain the battle, but I also want to give you the keys to walking in freedom."

The battle that I believe Paul could be talking about is addictive behavior. Paul could be talking about sexual addiction or any type of addiction. Sexual addiction is just as real as drug addiction, and the battle begins in the mind. The mind is a fascinating tool, and that's where the enemy begins to attack. Of course, no one can see what is going on in your mind.

The Word of God has power to expose darkness and bring light, for light will drive out and destroy the darkness in your life.

The main battle is lust itself. Lust is the nature that dwells in the soul. The only way lust can live on the inside of you is by feeding it. The way it lives is through the imagination, which produces what we call "fantasizing."

If you learn to harness your imagination and focus your imagination, it can produce freedom. "Focus" means to adjust the lens to produce a clear image. But if your imagination is not focused, if you are fantasizing, imagining, or indulging in things that are not real, they will produce bondage on the inside of you. The more you feed, the more you fantasize. But once you focus the imagination and learn to control it, it will produce freedom.

IF YOU LEARN TO HARNESS YOUR IMAGINATION AND FOCUS YOUR IMAGINATION, IT CAN PRODUCE FREEDOM.

Seven Ways to Open the Door to Sexual Addiction

Let me identify seven things that will open the door to sexual addiction:

1. Sexual addiction sometimes begins in men or young boys by the rejection of their father.

I'm not here to give you a sad story, and I'm not here to hear your sad story, but I am here to tell you, fathers, let's become fathers. Let's be better fathers. Let's not make our children pay for what our fathers did not do for us.

Paul found Timothy as a young man, and Timothy was a half-breed; He was half one nationality and half another. He didn't have a place to fit in. Paul said, "I'm going to be your spiritual father and I'm going to mentor you. I'm going to minister to you and I'm going to train you."

2. Many times sexual addictions begin by molestation or incest.

Molestation doesn't just happen to young girls. Young boys are molested too. One in three girls and one in six boys are sexually abused before the age of eighteen.[2]

A survey of high school adolescents showed that 17 percent of girls were physically abused and 12 percent were sexually abused, while 12 percent of boys were physically abused and 5 percent were sexually abused.[3]

The Women's Safety Project survey reported the following results regarding child abuse.[4]

- 17% of women reported at least one unwanted sexual contact (narrowly defined) by a relative before the age of 16. This suggests that approximately 1 in 6 girls have been sexually abused by a relative in childhood.

- 34% of women reported at least one unwanted sexual contact by a non-relative before age 16, suggesting that 1 in 3 girls is sexually abused by a non-relative in childhood.
- In total, 42% of women reported at least one experience of incestuous and/or extra familial sexual abuse before the age of 16. 27% were sexually abused before age 8.

- If a broader definition is used, including unwanted kisses, non-genital sexual touching, or non-contact experiences such as having someone masturbate in front of them, 53.8% of women reported an unwanted sexual experience before age 16.

Four-and-a-half percent (4.5%) of women report an incestuous experience with a father or stepfather before the age of 18. Girls with stepfathers are seven times more likely to be sexually abused than other girls. Of girls with biological fathers, 2.3% are sexually abused. Seventeen percent (17%) of girls with stepfathers are sexually abused by them.[5]

Four point nine percent (4.9%) of women report an incestuous experience with an uncle before the age of 18.[6]

Two percent (2%) of women report an incestuous experience with a brother.[7]

Sexual abuse in childhood usually creates emotional and psychological problems that last into adulthood. Incest may cause even greater harm because of the betrayal and the complications of the close personal relationship.

3. Sexual addictions are formed through pornography.

The majority of all *adult* magazines end up in the hands of teenagers or young children.

SEXUAL ABUSE IN CHILDHOOD USUALLY CREATES EMOTIONAL AND PSYCHOLOGICAL PROBLEMS THAT LAST INTO ADULTHOOD.

When I was a young boy, my dad was in the Air Force. I can remember coming back from Hawaii with my mother when my parents were breaking up. We had to live with my grandmother. At the time, she had a lot of sons living at home and maybe a couple of daughters. We all lived in a three-bedroom house with only one bath! I can remember going out back and walking on a trail through the woods to the store to buy a Coke or candy. I remember finding a magazine on that dirt trail that had pornography in it. In those days, pornography didn't look like it does today. Women's eyes were blocked out. I was only six or seven years old at the time, yet it ended up in my hands.

PORNOGRAPHY BRINGS SEXUAL ADDICTION.

The fact is, pornography is never destroyed or just thrown away; most of the time it ends up in the hands of the innocent. Pornography feeds a giant, a monster, on the inside of you. Pornography brings sexual addiction, and today we have the opportunity to visit sites on the Internet that are full of the most bizarre, vile garbage. There is a fight going on for our freedom today, and it's going to take accountability to walk in freedom.

4. Sexual addictions grow through fantasizing.

You can fantasize without even having sex. You can fantasize on the job or in a classroom. You can sit there and roll it over in your mind, and what you are doing is giving way to the enemy to continue to hold you in bondage.

THE VOICE OF FANTASIZING IN OUR MINDS IS AN AREA WE WANT TO CLOSE OFF.

The voice of fantasizing in our minds is an area we want to close off. The worst level of fantasizing is when you are having a sexual relationship with your wife and you are fantasizing about some other woman. That's a sexual addiction. Sometimes we think, *every man has it.* But our goal is not to be like every man. Our goal is to be like Jesus Christ. It's to be clean and free from sexual addiction.

5. Sexual addiction is fed through masturbation.

Most of the time when men are doing the "Big M," they are not thinking about their wife, they are thinking about other women. To be aroused, you have to use your imagination.

The "Big M" is a trap that opens the door and feeds all types of lust. Self-control, on the other hand, is a work of the Holy Spirit. As you yield to Him and ask Him to strengthen you in your weakness, He will reveal

God's Word that gives you power to resist the "Big M" at the moment of thoughts about it.

6. Sexual addiction is fed through calling 900 numbers: sex talk, dirty talk, and nasty talk.

People find themselves trapped in sexual addictions not knowing how to get out. The enemy uses fantasy to rob us of reality, and some of the forms that people are trapped in is the industry of 900 numbers.

Sexual addiction is like any other compulsive lifestyle. Most sexual addictions go unnoticed, leaving those trapped by the lies they believe, or masking their guilt and fear, swimming in a pool of self-pity.

7. Sexual addiction is fed through immoral relationships.

We want to stop immoral relationships from happening in your life before they occur. This is pre-game talk! I am trying to build a winning team, and we have to get down to brass tacks to have a winning team. God wants you on this winning team – the National Freedom League! So we've got to have coaches and assistants. To do this, we have to be able to talk from gut level of what is going on in men's lives.

Five Areas of Immoral Relationships

There are five areas of immoral relationships. We will look briefly at each of these areas:

1. Adultery.

The Bible says that sin is fun for a season, but it will cost you. It will make you pay more than you want to pay, it will take you further than you want to go, and it will make you stay longer than you want to stay.

2. Fornication.

There is a difference between adultery and fornication. The simplest definition for fornication is that it is any immorality or sexual relationship between people who are not married; adultery is between married people.

3. Prostitution.

Many movies have prostitution in them, and it causes men to think, *Wouldn't that be great to go down and buy a piece one time and see what it's like?* You will end up with a disease or with something you are going to take home to your wife.

Solomon said it's more than a disease. He said in Proverbs 5:9 that you are going to give away your honor. In Proverbs 5:3 Solomon gives a warning about the strange woman: **"For the lips of a strange woman drop as an honeycomb. . . ."**

When you approach the strange woman – the prostitute – she is only after one thing: payday! She is going to tell you, "You look good. You are a hunk, a fine guy. I'm going to satisfy you." She is lying! Why? Because **"her mouth is smoother than oil: but her end is bitter as wormwood . . ."** (Proverbs 5:3-4).

At one time I heard a teaching on "wormwood." Dake's Bible defines "wormwood," as "a plant of which there are several species, all being distinguished for intense bitterness and some being very harmful." Vine, Unger, and White define "wormwood" in the Greek as "a plant both bitter and deleterious, and growing in desolate places, figuratively suggestive of 'calamity' and 'injustice.'"[8]

THERE IS SOMETHING WORSE THAN DYING, AND THAT IS LIVING YOUR LIFE WITHOUT HONOR.

Solomon continues to describe the strange woman:

Her feet go down to death; her steps take hold on hell . . .

Remove thy way far from her, and come not nigh the door of her house:

Lest thou give thine honour unto others. . . .

Proverbs 5:5,8-9

You don't want to lose your honor. There is something worse than dying, and that is living your life without honor.

Proverbs 5:15 says, **"Drink waters out of thine own cistern. . . ."** A cistern is a water pool, a holding spot. The Bible tells you that's where you drink your water – from your own spouse.

Verses 18 and 19 say:

Let thy fountain be blessed: and rejoice with the wife of thy youth.

> **Let her be as the loving hind and pleasant roe; let her breasts satisfy thee at all times; and be thou ravished always with her love.**

Solomon is talking about married people. He is always warning about the "strange woman" and how she has power over you once you yield to her seduction. Once she gains power over you, you cannot break free automatically.

4. Homosexuality

This is a sexual relationship between two men. The *Amplified Bible* says in First Corinthians 6:9: "**Do you not know that the unrighteous and the wrongdoers will not inherit or have any share in the kingdom of God? Do not be deceived (misled): neither the impure and immoral, nor idolaters, nor adulterers, nor those who participate in homosexuality**"

Homosexuality in the Greek is the word "uncleanness." Greek: *akatharsia,* whatever is opposite of purity; including sodomy, homosexuality, lesbianism, pederasty, and all other forms of sexual perversion. (Reference verses: Galatians 5:19; Matthew 23:27; Romans 1:21-32, 6:19; 2 Corinthians 12:21; Ephesians 4:19; 5:3; Colossians 3:5; 1 Thessalonians 2:3; 4:7; 2 Peter 2).[9]

5. Bestiality

Leviticus 20:15 says, **"And if a man lie with a beast, he shall surely be put to death; and ye shall slay the beast."**

Dake said in his footnotes of Leviticus 20:15:

Bestiality (sexual relations with a beast) has been practiced in pagan nations by both men and women. For this and other sins the Canaanites were destroyed (Leviticus 18:19-25, 20:22-24). Describing sexual relations between men and women, the Bible says they become one flesh, even in harlotry (2 Corinthians 6:15-18). Bestiality thus reduces man, who was made in the image of God, to becoming one flesh with a beast! Hence, it insults the Creator more than some other sins. It was God's plan for man to be higher in morals and principles than to cohabit with senseless dumb animals. Just as murder is a serious crime against God because it takes the life of one created in His image (Genesis 9:6), so bestiality lowers one of His likeness to the level of a beast. For this sin both the person and the beast were to be killed, though the beast had no moral responsibility.[10]

How to Overcome

The Bible teaches us plainly how to overcome. Let's read Second Corinthians 10:4-5:

> **(For the weapons of our warfare are not carnal, but mighty through God to the pulling down of strong holds;)**
>
> **Casting down imaginations. . . .**

You can insert the word "fantasizing" for the word "imaginations" since that is where addictive behaviors begin. Verse 5 in *The Amplified Version* says, **"argu-**

ments." First of all, it's an argument in your mind. The enemy tries to argue with you, and there is an argument going on. It's not a war yet.

THERE IS A ROAD IN YOUR MIND THAT CAN LEAD YOU TO THE RIGHT PLACE OR TO THE WRONG PLACE.

There is a road in your mind that can lead you to the right place or to the wrong place. Who is going to win? The one who wins is the strongest one. If you feed lust, lust will win. But if you make a decision to shut the door on lust by not feeding it, you can win.

It's going to take more than a prayer line to help you. It's going to take more than anointing oil. It's going to take more than a deliverance service to win over lust. You've got to control your eyes and your thoughts.

The Three-Second Rule

When we had a guest speaker at one of our men's meetings, our guest taught us something that is very valuable called the "three-second rule." The "three-second rule" is when you see a girl or something inappropriate, for instance on television, you have three seconds to make up your mind and turn the other way.

THE "THREE-SECOND RULE" IS WHEN YOU SEE A GIRL OR SOMETHING INAPPROPRIATE, FOR INSTANCE ON TELEVISION, YOU HAVE THREE SECONDS TO MAKE UP YOUR MIND AND TURN THE OTHER WAY.

Our youth minister, Matt, and I were driving down the

road on a Saturday after we heard teaching on the "three-second rule." An old man pulled up on a motorcycle without a shirt on and he had big hooters hanging down with gray hair on his chest, and tattoos all over his body. I looked over and started laughing. Immediately Matt said, "Three-second rule!"

I found out that the "three-second rule" not only works with women. It works with anything that you shouldn't look at, any object that would divide your attention from purity.

The Bible teaches us, **"Casting down imaginations** [fantasizing]**, and every high thing** [arguments, theories, or reasonings] **that exalteth itself against the knowledge of God, and bringing into captivity every thought to the obedience of Christ"** (2 Corinthians 10:5).

This is how you win the battle – by bringing every thought captive, casting thoughts down. Jesus taught us to **"take no thought"** (Matthew 6:25). Jesus had some tough things to say about the mind. He said, **"But I say unto you, That whosoever looketh on a woman to lust after her hath committed adultery with her already in his heart"** (Matthew 5:28).

Some men say, "Well, I've already committed adultery with her in my heart, so I might as well go ahead and do it physically." Not so! Jesus is teaching you to stop before it becomes adultery in your heart.

There is a reason why you should not commit the act of adultery. I want to show you what Paul said about it.

He lets us know that something else is going to happen to you: **"Flee fornication. Every sin that a man doeth is without the body; but he that commiteth fornication sinneth against his own body"** (1 Corinthians 6:18). He said, "You are sinning against your own body." Really what he is saying is, "You are breaking down your resistance to stand against sin."

I've had men who have committed fornication or adultery say to me, "I'll never do it again." But unless the following five areas are strengthened in their character, they will do it again:

- Loyalty
- Faithfulness
- Honesty
- Dependability
- Commitment

We want to be loyal, faithful, honest, dependable, and committed men who walk after God and walk in agreement with His Word. This is the type of men we want to be.

IF YOU HAVE LOST YOUR HONOR, YOU CAN REGAIN IT, BUT YOU WILL NEVER REGAIN IT BY YOURSELF.

If you have lost your honor, you can regain it, but you will never regain it by yourself. It's going to take a team of men working together – men who will support and encourage one another and hold each other accountable!

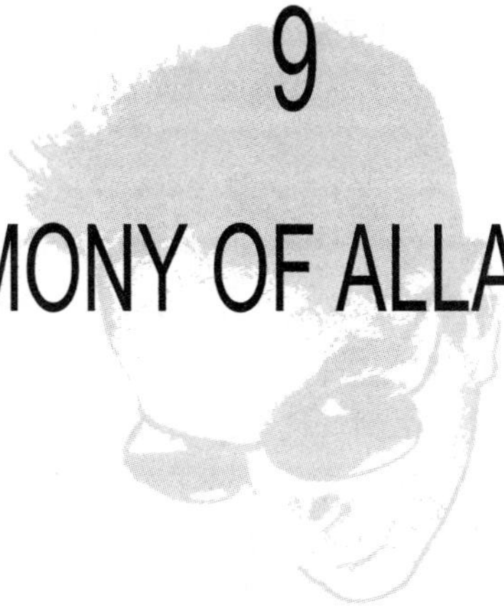

9

TESTIMONY OF ALLAN SEALS

I would like for you to open up your Bibles to a key scripture that speaks about our freedom from bondages. Before I get into my testimony of what God has done for me let's read this key scripture.

> **But he was wounded for our transgressions, he was bruised for our iniquities....**
>
> **Isaiah 53:5**

A "transgression" is a sin, while an "iniquity" is a bruise. A bruise is inner, and a wound is outer. So what's the difference between "iniquities" and "transgressions"? A "transgression" could be a one- or two-time thing, but an "iniquity" is a habitual thing. An "iniquity" is something that comes inside of your innermost being and controls you.

AN "INIQUITY" IS SOMETHING THAT COMES INSIDE OF YOUR INNERMOST BEING AND CONTROLS YOU.

I spent twenty-eight years of my life bound by sexual addiction. I was tormented and Satan had me on a yo-yo, up and down.

Once I was set free of sexual addiction, I had a group called "Pure Life Ministries." We ministered to over two hundred men in a church and probably another fifty or sixty men at the Correctional Center in Missouri. We found that most of the men didn't know that they were hooked by little sins.

Satan wants to hook you, so you start out with a small sin and there's a hook in it. All sin is pleasurable for a season or we wouldn't do it. It's important to know that what may seem pleasurable for a moment has a hook in it if God says not to do it.

I was delivered from being a sex addict more than twelve years ago. I realized that it's real easy to stay out of sin if you know how to do it. If you are tempted and you know to stay away from temptation, it's pretty simple.

But why isn't it that simple for most? I found the answer really is in your relationship with the Lord. The closer I am to the Lord, the less I want to sin.

I was born again in 1975. Even as a Christian, I was in sexual addiction, but I didn't have a close relationship with the Lord.

The Word says, **"Ye shall seek me, and find me, when ye shall search for me with all your heart. And I will be found of you, saith the Lord...."**

(Jeremiah 29:13-14). If you will get close to the Lord, He will get close to you. (See James 4:8.) As I drew closer to the Lord, my desire to sin was less and less. So it's easy for me now as a past sex addict to say, "How do you keep from doing it?" You get close to God. That's the answer!

If you are real honest with yourself, you commit sin in secret because you don't believe God is watching you. You think, *If my wife doesn't catch me or my sons, my brother, my mother or father, or whoever doesn't catch me, I am free and clear.*

That's a lie, because God is omnipresent and He sees everything that is going on. If you have a relationship with God and you know He is watching you, that fear of God, which is the beginning of wisdom, will keep you from sinning. So you need to look at your relationship with God, because if you are closing Him out and sinning anyway, then your relationship with Him is in dire need of restoration.

IF YOU DON'T HAVE LOVE FROM A PHYSICAL FATHER, THERE IS A VOID.

Pastor Brian talked about how rejection can actually start sexual addiction. That's what happened in my case. I had a stepfather who didn't give a flip about me or my sister and I never met my real father. So immediately it was a setup for rejection, because we didn't have any love. When you don't receive love from a physical father, it is hard to accept love from a spiritual father. If you don't have love from a physical father, there is a void. All of us were created to be loved and when your father doesn't fill that love for you, you are going to fill it with something else.

I even believe that when you are in your mother's womb, if there is rejection – you appear to be an accident and your mother and father don't want you – the spirit in the womb can pick up that rejection. Also, you can experience rejection at birth as well as when you are growing up.

I was rejected as a kid. My mother abandoned my sister and me to go on a trip with my stepdad who was a truck driver.

So when I was about fifteen, I started looking at pornography. My grandfather lived with us and he had some books, which he hid under his mattress.

I have told men who have gone through the Pure Life Ministries Program, "If you have pornography in a book in your house, I guarantee you that your kids will find it no matter where you put it. You need to get it out of your house, and if you think it's in a safe place, you are deceived."

So I started with pornography and it was filling the void in my life. It was giving me pleasure that I didn't receive from anything else, so I was filling that gap. And of course, like anything, whether it's drugs or alcohol, you take a little and all of a sudden that becomes mundane or normal and you want something a little more exciting. So you go from the *Playboy* or other such magazines into hard-core pornography. That's what I got into.

This opened me up to being lustful as a teenager. I was molested by a man when I was fifteen. When that happened, the first thing I thought was, *Am I going to turn out to be a homosexual?* That grated on me for years and kept me on a spiral of degradation as I got into homosexuality and pornography. That went on until I graduated. Then, I thought, *I'm going to join the Air Force, become a man, get rid of this thing, and be done with it.*

I joined the Air Force and got married. I thought getting married would help solve the pornography problem and the desire for lust, but that was a lie.

WHEN YOU GET IN SEXUAL ADDICTION, NORMAL SEX DOESN'T SATISFY.

I had been married for two years when I was sent to Greenland. There are no women in Greenland, so what do men do in Greenland but watch pornography. I mean, we had officers who would come and watch pornography films with us, so we thought it was no big deal, yet it was feeding that spiral of degradation.

After seven years of marriage and two children, my first marriage ended in a divorce because I wasn't satisfied with normal sex. When you get in sexual addiction, normal sex doesn't satisfy. That's why you have to be careful of pornography and why it has such a hook. It will drive you like drugs to accept it and you think, *It's no big deal. No one sees I'm doing it and no one cares I'm doing it.* But what you are taking in is a poison that you won't be able to deliver yourself out of.

My rationale for the divorce was, "I must not love my wife because I had an affair, so we might as well not stay together. We are arguing and fighting all the time, so it's best for the kids if we separate."

I started the same thing with my kids that my father did with me. He wasn't there, so what I thought was good for the kids really was a selfish thing. I wanted to continue to do my thing and have my kids around too. We fought for the kids and I put on a show that I wanted them, but I didn't get them.

I lost my job, I went through bankruptcy, I lost my wife and my children, and I lost my integrity and self-esteem. I lost everything and I was at the bottom of the pit. That's when I accepted Jesus Christ as my Lord. Many of us do that when we're at the bottom!

I met another girl in a bar, and we decided to get married. After two years of marriage, things started going downhill. Finally, after four years of marriage and one daughter, we decided to break up because we just weren't getting along and it was a mutual thing. She wasn't happy with me and I wasn't happy with her.

The same thread that went through this relationship was, you are never satisfied with what you have, because pornography instills pictures of what you want and desire. I always felt I deserved better, which is another lie, and I always felt I could do better, which is another lie.

After that marriage, I started to give up on marriage. Then I thought, *Maybe if I meet a Christian girl instead of someone at the bar, this will solve my problem.*

I met a Christian girl who became my third wife, and it lasted for two years. The same problem came up again and we broke it off and separated. I didn't know what was going on. I didn't have the answers. I knew I had this problem, but I didn't know what it was and I didn't know why it was tearing me up.

I always blamed the women. I thought they were the big problem. They weren't satisfying my needs, so it was their problem, not mine. I had these weird ideas of satisfying me – ideas I got from pornography.

I read some information from a doctor who said that when you see certain things and you have a climax when you are watching pornography, it puts photographs in your mind permanently. When you climax at the time you are looking at porn, then what happens is that's what is needed to trigger it every time. So if you are looking at pornography and you climax, that is the only thing that will stimulate you.

Because I was "experienced" with marriage failures, I went to a Divorce Recovery class where I was welcomed with open arms. This is when I met my present wife, Phyllis. We weren't in love with each other, but we were good friends. We got married and it only lasted three years. Problems started arising again. I told Phyllis it just wasn't working, so we separated. She didn't want it, but I felt that it wasn't working so I planned to file for divorce.

Our marriage hung by a string, but sometimes that's all God needs. One night I called Phyllis over to my place and we sat down and talked. I thought, *I'm just going to be honest with her.*

The sexual sin I was in was so horrendous, I had never been able to tell any of my wives. I was never able to tell my sister or my brother and I couldn't tell my mother. I couldn't tell my pastor and I couldn't even tell my best friend.

When you get into pornography, that causes you to get into other things, whether it's group sex or going to the bars and picking up a person you don't even know and having sex with them. When you start doing things like that, you lose reality. So I thought, *I'm just going to lay it on the line and tell Phyllis.*

I remember her sitting at the table as I opened my heart up to her. I said, "Phyllis, I'm just going to be honest with you. Here is what I have been through. I don't know why I am having a problem, but these are some of the things I have done. I hate unloading this on you, but I feel like I need to."

What I expected her to do was get up and walk out, call me a few names, and that would be it, but something miraculous happened. She looked at me and said, "Allan, I hate the sin that you have been in, but I love you." That was the first time in my life that I ever felt God's love directed to me because I was never able to accept God's love, even as a born-again Christian. But when her love came through when she said, "Allan, I love you no matter what you have done; I hate the sin you are in, but I love you," I was blown apart! Then it was like God saying, "And that's how I love you. I hate the sin you are in, but I love you!"

When I told Phyllis that, I decided to get some help. Shortly after that, I heard Dr. Dobson talking about a guy who had Pure Life Ministries and talking about how he was in sexual addiction because of pornography. He was an ex-policeman and he was picking up prostitutes and doing all kinds of things.

I ordered Dr. Dobson's tapes and listened to them. I thought, *What's this, "sexual addiction"?* I had never heard that, but I found out that's what I was in. I was addicted to sex and I was miserable. I had to admit it like a drug addict or an alcoholic. I had to get help and I needed a way to get out of it. My sexual triggers, as well as what to avoid, were identified.

Some people claim that homosexuality is a disease, but that is a lie of the devil. It is sin, so you can repent, turn from it, and be free of it.

I decided that I would do anything to get rid of the sexual addiction. You have to be at a point that you are so disgusted with it that you want to get rid of it.

Now, I have had men come through Pure Life Ministries say, "I don't think I want to get rid of it." I mean, these are men who are cheating on their wives and dealing with pornography. They aren't ready to give it up so they keep on doing it.

One thing about it, if you get hooked on pornography and it takes you down the road until you get addicted to it, you are going to wind up dead; you'll have HIV; you will wind up in jail; or you will lose your job and your family. There are no other alternatives. That's what you are looking at. That's what happens to people who are addicted to sex, because they have no control. It is iniquity and you have no control to stop it in yourself. Until you get so tired of it ruling your life and you decide to go the opposite direction, getting closer to God and building a relationship with Him, you will never change.

Some of the things I had to avoid were skin and R-rated TV programs. You have to be selective of the kind of music you listen to, because some music has sexual, demonic beats. Some of the bands are demonically controlled and their music just carries it on. Also, you have to watch the magazines that come to your house and get rid of those that are sexually implicit.

None of us as men want our wives to tell us what to do, but they can be a big helpmate. I hated it when my wife came in the living room and said, "Allan, you shouldn't be watching that program." I thought, *You're not the Holy Spirit!*

My attitude should have been, "You are right." Click! Shut it off. But it's pride or arrogance that causes us as men not to want to be told what to do, so I advise the wives, be gentle about it.

I visited porn shops and went to bookstores, even as a Christian. You think, *Why is a Christian guy tied up in that?* Because this addiction is so hard to get free from.

You have two natures. Before you were born again, you had an old nature. When you were born again, you received a new nature. That old nature is dead, but you can keep it alive if you don't put it to death by not feeding it. Paul said, **"I die daily."** You have to put that old nature in your mind to death. If you have a new nature in your spirit and an old nature in your mind, which one are you feeding? If you are feeding the old nature in your mind and imagination, it is going to play war with you every day.

If you will feed your new nature the Word of God, it will grow. Whichever nature you feed is the one that will consume your life. If you are in the Word daily, if you are going to church regularly, if you are seeking God, and if you are praying, then you are feeding your new nature and the old nature is going to die. It will be so dead it will no longer have any effect on you.

There are certain things you know you can't afford to do, so develop a plan to overcome your addiction. If you don't have a plan, you will go by your gland! Who wants to be led by their gland?

If you are in any type of sin, repent, turn from it, and seek God. That will keep you from staying in it.

Comments from Pastor Brian

I appreciate Allan for being honest, frank, and upfront with us, because I think we have tiptoed around this subject for years. We didn't want to bring it up in the church because it makes people uncomfortable, but failure and losing your integrity will make you feel even more uncomfortable. The reason Allan has shared with us is we don't want to lose our honor.

The basic thing I see for you to be sexually addicted and to remain addicted is for you to feed it. So you need to identify what is feeding it and make a commitment to shut off whatever is feeding the wrong desires in your life.

The Blood of Jesus

The blood of Jesus Christ is what does the cleansing. Hebrews 9:14 says, **"How much more shall the blood of Christ, who through the eternal Spirit offered himself without spot to God, purge your conscience from dead works to serve the living God?"** The blood purges your conscience from dead works.

At first I didn't understand what this was talking about and I began to look at different translations. *The New English Bible* says, **"Cleanses our conscience from the deadness of our former ways."** So speaking the blood and confessing the blood will go into your conscience and cleanse you.

The iniquity of sexual sins is tattooed in your soul. A tattoo to your soul is more painful to be removed than removing a tattoo from your skin.

There is one thing that has the ability to remove that from your soul, and that is the blood of Jesus Christ. You have to be proactive if you want to change. What I mean by proactive is you have to hate your iniquity. Hebrews 1:9 says, **"Thou hast loved righteousness, and hated iniquity. . . ."** You have to hate the iniquity that's on the inside of you, you have to be proactive, and you have to make some commitments to be cleansed.

THE BLOOD, CONFESSION OF THE WORD, AND HONESTY WILL SET YOU FREE AND KEEP YOU FREE FROM GOING BACK INTO SEXUAL ADDICTION.

The blood, confession of the Word, and honesty will set you free and keep you free from going back into sexual addiction.

You have to come to the place that Allan spoke about and that is to accept the love of God and His forgiveness. God loves you, Jesus loves you, and I love you. We need to express our love for one another. It's not a gay thing as a man to tell another man that you love him in the Lord. We need to have love for one another.

10

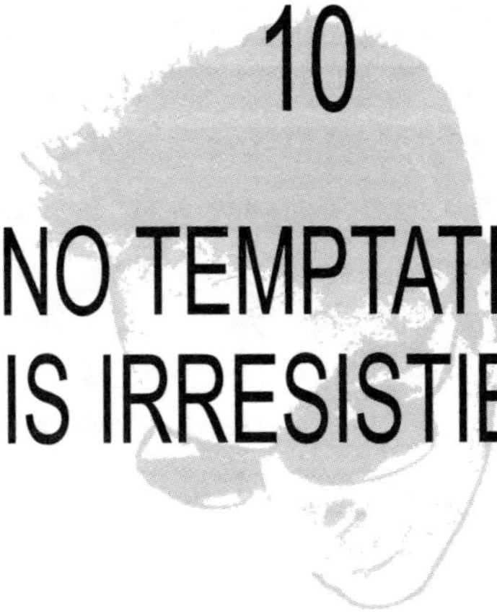

NO TEMPTATION IS IRRESISTIBLE

First Corinthians 10:13 says, **"There hath no temptation taken you but such as is common to man: but God is faithful, who will not suffer you to be tempted above that ye are able; but will with the temptation also make a way to escape, that ye may be able to bear it."**

This scripture is not saying what many preachers say it says. Many preachers share this scripture and they only know one thing about it. That is, "God will not put more on you than you are able to bear." That is not what this scripture is saying. God does not put anything on you anyhow! God wants to free you.

What this scripture is saying is,

1. There is no temptation that is irresistible, meaning there is no temptation you cannot resist.
2. Every temptation has a limitation in its power and time.
3. God has set the rules that He will not allow you to be tempted beyond what you can bear.

As you read the *Amplified Translation* of this scripture, you will see more clearly God's plan for your life and how God will not leave you in the middle of the temptation. But I must make this note also, that if you yield yourself to viewing porn or lustful magazines, lust will rise up and control you.

The Amplified says: **"For no temptation (no trial regarded as enticing to sin, no matter how it comes or where it leads) has overtaken you and laid hold on you that is not common to man [that is, no temptation or trial has come to you that is beyond human resistance and that is not adjusted and adapted and belonging to human experience, and such as man can bear]. But God is faithful [to His Word and to His compassionate nature], and He [can be trusted] not to let you be tempted and tried and assayed beyond your ability and strength of resistance and power to endure, but with the temptation He will [always] also provide the way out (the means of escape to a landing place), that you may be capable and strong and powerful to bear up under it patiently."**

You can win over every temptation that comes your way when you are an honest man, a submitted man, a man of honor, and a man who has the Word abiding in him.

> SECRETS WILL KEEP PEOPLE SICK. GOD HEALS WHAT YOU REVEAL.

Secrets will keep people sick. God heals what you reveal. He wants to heal you if you have been sexually abused. You have to understand that many times sexual abuse leads to sexual addictions. Today many people are bound by sexual addictions and even if you were or were not abused when you were a child, you need to understand that addictions cannot rule your life if you do not yield to them.

You must drag sexual addiction by its neck into the light of the Word of God. Overcoming the fear of what other people will think about you when you drag it into the light is most of the battle of winning over it, because it's no longer hidden on the inside of your soul. You must make up your mind that you are not going to feed it any longer through your eyes, but you are going to guard your eyes.

Most people believe that there should be modesty in the way women dress. But what if they never dress the way you think they ought to dress? As men, we ought to rise above it and control our thoughts. We should not walk around saying, "How do you expect me not to look?" The problem is, it's not just the look. It's what happens when the gaze starts.

IT IS WHAT YOU SEE THAT WILL TRIGGER LUST ON THE INSIDE OF YOU.

In Matthew 5:28 Jesus said, **"Whosoever looketh on a woman to lust after her hath committed adultery with her already in his heart."** The word for "looketh" is to look at, to set a gaze, with wide-open eyes. <u>At the moment of the</u>

thought, it is not a sin, but if you lust in your heart, it is equal to adultery.

In the first epistle of John, he compares hating your brother to murder. So where do we stop the rat race? We stop it by realizing we have power over our eyesight. Remember when blinders were put on the side of a mule's eyes so he would look a certain direction? As men, we need these blinders or new boundaries for our minds!

It is what you see that will trigger lust on the inside of you. When you get up in the morning, make your mind up, "I am going to control my eyes." Then test yourself every fifteen minutes throughout the day. When you see something provocative, say, "No, I resist you in the name of Jesus." Say to yourself, "Lady Lust and the red lizard do NOT have power over me."

This brings us back to our teaching on the "three-second rule," meaning that you have three seconds to turn and look the other way!

Men's eyes are automatically drawn to the breast and to the rear, so learn to control your eyes, your thoughts, and your imagination. Ask God to remove the iniquity that causes you to fantasize. That is the renewing of the mind process, which will reverse destructive habits and iniquity in your life. Your spirit is well able to master your soul, which includes your mind and imagination.

YOUR SPIRIT IS WELL ABLE TO MASTER YOUR SOUL, WHICH INCLUDES YOUR MIND AND IMAGINATION.

We need not only to understand the anatomy of a man, but the total spiritual psychology of man that Paul declared in First Thessalonians 5:23, that man is a three-part being. Paul is not saying what psychology tells us – that man is a mind and a body. Paul is saying by the Spirit of God that man is a spirit, like God. He can be king over his mind, thoughts, flesh, Lady Lust, and the red lizard as he feeds upon the Word of God and meditates upon it.

FANTASIZING IS NOTHING MORE THAN MEDITATING ON WRONG THINGS UNTIL THEY BECOME ALIVE ON THE INSIDE OF YOU.

Fantasizing

Fantasizing is nothing more than meditating on wrong things until they become alive on the inside of you. Fantasizing causes perversion to grow and it ruins your relationships. The next thing you know, your bed is defiled.

Lust will not die on the inside of you just because you get married. When a man gets married, the first thing that comes to his mind is, "Now I can have sex as much as I want when I want it." You will find out real quick that's an unrealistic expectation!

The "Big M" is not just a problem of your teenage years. That habit can be carried right into your married life because it's such an easy way to escape the pressure that builds up on the inside of you.

11

BECOMING A MAN OF HONOR

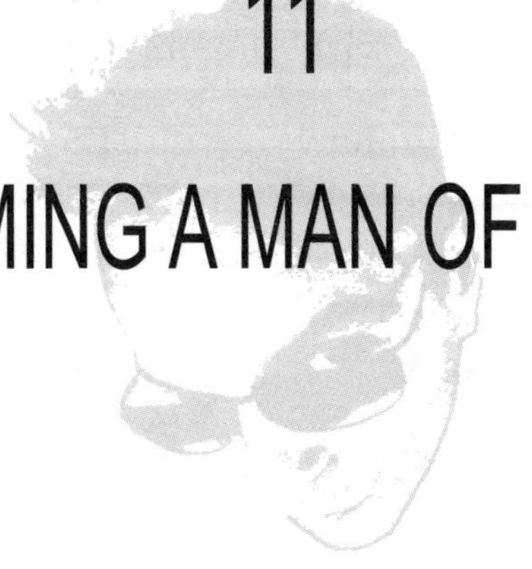

There is only one thing that is worse than dying and that is living without honor. God wants you to be a man of honor.

There are four keys to becoming a man of honor:

1. **To be a man of honor, you must honor the Holy Spirit in your life.** [The Holy Spirit wants to mentor you.]

To be a man of honor or to regain your honor you must be a follower of the Word of God and allow the Holy Spirit to be your mentor. One of the first areas that He will lead you into is a life of purity. (John 16:8-15.)

God asks you to humble yourself, to be honest with yourself, and to seek help from someone who has the knowledge to assist you to walk in freedom. (Proverbs 15:33.)

2. **To be a man of honor, you must honor the Lord with your substance and the first-**

fruits of all your increase. [This means to honor the Lord with your money.]

To be a man of honor you must not be a lover of money, you must become a master of money. As you honor God with your money by giving Him your firstfruits, God will honor you. (Proverbs 3:9-10.)

> TO BE A MAN OF HONOR YOU MUST NOT BE A LOVER OF MONEY, YOU MUST BECOME A MASTER OF MONEY.

Many people are in bondage to the lust of money. Money is one of the three evils [sex, money, and power] that the red lizard tries to get us to seek and sell our soul out to.

What God wanted to do in you, He did in Christ. You are a God-made man of wealth who is able to bless others and support the work of God. As we keep the covenant of God, we release the blessing on our lives and the lives of our families. As a man of honor, you put God first and you support your family. You don't run off with another man's wife and leave your kids to be raised by your wife and not support them financially. You can't be a deadbeat dad and go around to meetings raising your hands and saying amen when you don't honor your obligations. When you become a man of honor, you will walk in the wisdom of God and the wealth of God will follow.

3. **To be a man of honor, you must honor those who are over you in the Lord.** [The Bible teaches us to submit to those who are in authority over us.]

To be a man of honor, you have to be a man of submission. When the centurion came to the Lord, he said, "I am a man under authority," not a man in authority. A man who is under authority can have authority. Most men want to be in authority, but authority is given by God when we walk in submission to those He has placed in our lives.

The centurion said to Jesus: "Speak the word only. You don't have to come into my house. Your word is equal to Your person. Just speak Your word, because I see that You are a man in authority and I am going to get under Your authority. When I get under Your authority, Your power will flow through Your words right into my house to my servant." (See Matthew 8:5-13.)

MARRIAGE IS DESIGNED BY GOD TO REFLECT HIS GLORY AND MAN IS TO HONOR GOD BY HONORING HIS WIFE.

The Bible tells us that if we submit unto God, we can resist the devil and he will flee. (See James 4:7.) The Bible teaches us to submit to our leaders. (See Hebrews 13:17.)

4. **To be a man of honor, you must honor your wife. If you honor your wife, God will honor you.**

To be a man of honor you must honor your wife and love her the same way Christ loves the Church. Most men are selfish and rebellious, but the God-made man is a man created after God in His image.

Marriage is designed by God to reflect His glory and man is to honor God by honoring his wife. The Bible tells us that our prayers can be hindered if we do not honor our wives. The Bible also teaches us that we should leave our father and mother and cleave to our wife. "Leave" means to break the ties. "Cleave" means to pursue after her and look towards her for your emotional support.

"Leave" and "cleave" are good things to remember. "Cleave" also means to show passion and romance to your wife. Her desire is for a man who will serve God and show her the passion and love that she desires.

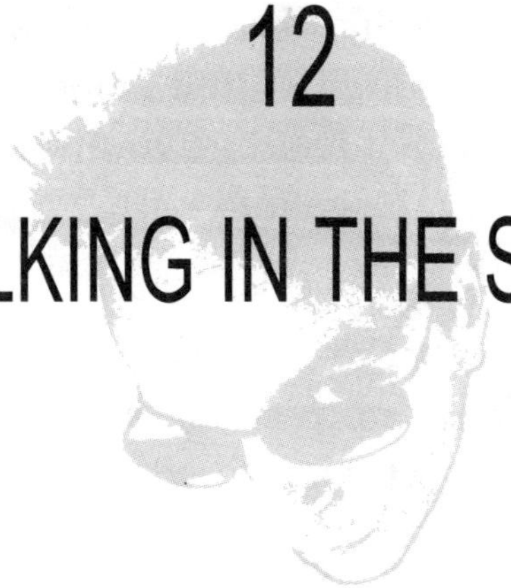

12

WALKING IN THE SPIRIT

This I say then, Walk in the Spirit, and ye shall not fulfil the lust of the flesh.

Galatians 5:16

And they that are Christ's have crucified the flesh with the affections and lusts.

Galatians 5:24

Paul, by the Spirit of God, gives us the key to overcoming the lust of the flesh with one simple phrase: "Walk in the Spirit." As we walk in the Spirit, we will not fulfill the lust of the flesh.

In First Thessalonians 5:23 Paul says, **"And the very God of peace sanctify you wholly; and I pray God your whole spirit and soul and body be preserved blameless unto the coming of our Lord Jesus Christ."**

When the Bible says to walk in the Spirit, it is saying to allow the Holy Spirit to take control of your life – every area of your life. Your spirit is the part of man with which you contact the realm of the Spirit; your soul is your mind, thoughts, and emotions with which you contact the world of feelings; and your body is your outer man that we can see and with which you contact this natural world.

The Holy Spirit is the God-Agent on earth today to empower you to walk in freedom, and He lives in your spirit. The phrases, "staying filled with the Spirit" and "walking in the Spirit" are speaking of the same thing. For you to live victoriously over the flesh, you have to stay filled with the Spirit.

Praying in the spirit allows you to become aware of the things of the Spirit of God. As you pray in the spirit, it is the Holy Spirit praying through you. Paul said, **"I will pray with the spirit, and I will pray with the understanding..."** (1 Corinthians 14:15). To pray with your spirit is to pray in your spiritual prayer language. To pray with your understanding is to pray with the human language that you know. Most people get in trouble the longer they pray in their native tongue. My native language is English and I mess it up all the time. People who get into doubt in their native language are speaking words of doubt every day.

WHATEVER THOUGHT YOU ALLOW TO LIVE IN YOUR MIND, YOU WILL BECOME A SERVANT OF THAT THOUGHT.

To walk in the Spirit, you have to spend time praying with your spirit. Then you will be able to walk victoriously over the lust of the flesh. Paul gives a detailed list of the things called "the works of the flesh." (See Galatians 5:19-21.) Another way to overcome the works of the flesh and to walk in the Spirit is to sit under the teaching of the Word of God. You will never rise to the place that God wants you to be at if you do not hear the Word of God. Whatever you hear the most will influence your life.

Scripture says, **"To whom ye yield yourselves servants to obey, his servants ye are to whom ye obey . . ."** (Romans 6:16). Whatever thought you allow to live in your mind, you will become a servant of that thought.

Hearing the Word of God is the beginning of the new things that God has for you. As you hear and meditate upon the Word of God, you will be able to see yourself the way God sees you right now – not weak and little but strong and mighty! Meditating upon God's Word daily will implant the seed of power within your life.

AS YOU MEDIATE UPON THE SCRIPTURES THAT REVEAL WHO YOU ARE IN CHRIST, THEN YOUR DESIRES WILL CHANGE BECAUSE OF THE ENGRAFTED WORD OF GOD WHICH ABIDES IN YOU.

To yield to the flesh, you must first think about it and meditate upon it. Then desire will rise up in you to produce an action. The flesh will try to get you to live out what you view in your imagination. You sow to your flesh and imagination by thinking and watching things that you should not think upon or watch.

Galatians 6:8 says, **"For he that soweth to his flesh shall of the flesh reap corruption; but he that soweth to the Spirit shall of the Spirit reap life everlasting."**

It's the same way with God's Word. As you meditate upon the scriptures that reveal who you are in Christ, then your desires will change because of the engrafted Word of God which abides in you. His Word living in you will cause your actions to change. Not only will His Word change your actions, but it will change your personality. The Word living in you will change your attitude about life and yourself. You will begin to see yourself the way God sees you. His image of you will rise in you and drive out things in you that are shameful.

Your actions will change by feeding upon the Word of God. Your mind is in the process of being renewed by changing what you are meditating upon. In Ephesians 5:18-19, the Holy Spirit gives us the key to walking in victory over the lust of the flesh: **"Be not drunk with wine . . . but be filled with the Spirit"** (v. 18). How? By **"speaking to yourselves in psalms and hymns and spiritual songs, singing and making melody in your heart to the Lord"** (v. 19). You have to speak to yourself every day to walk in freedom over the lust of the flesh.

Faith Declarations

Following is a list of faith declarations that you need to speak aloud over yourself and meditate upon every day:

Power Over Lust

Say this morning, noon, and night: *Today I will walk in freedom over lust. I speak to lust and command it to be broken off of my life because I am born of God and I am a son of God. Today I will guard my eyes to view and see those things that are pleasing to my Father. I refuse to look at and watch those things that build lust in my life. I will not look or gaze upon a woman to lust after her. I will quickly turn my head the other way and train my eyes to view the things that please my Father.*

Power Over My Imagination

Today I will control my thoughts and imagination. I refuse to allow lustful thoughts and greed to dominate my mind. The moment they come to me, I will speak to them in the name of Jesus and tell them to leave my mind now. I say to lust and greed, you are not welcome in my life. My mind belongs to God, and it is no longer a home of evil thoughts.

Power Over Unclean Spirits

When the urge comes to watch, listen, and speak things that are lustful, say: *I speak to that unclean spirit and command it to leave my life in the name of*

Jesus and by the blood of Jesus. My mind belongs to God, and it is not the property of lust and greed in Jesus' name.

Power Over My Sleep

Before you go to sleep at night, go to your room and say: *I speak the blood of Jesus over this room and I command the evil spirits of lust and fear to leave now in Jesus' name. I speak the peace of God to my mind, and I say that my sleep will be sweet, because God gives to His beloved in their sleep. My night seasons belong to God and not to the lust of the flesh.*

Power Over My Thoughts

I am a new creature in Christ Jesus. Old things have passed away. Behold, all things have become new. Lust, greed, pride, and selfishness no longer have power over me. I am a God-made man. I am free and I have power over my flesh. (2 Corinthians 5:17.) *I have power over what I see with my eyes. I refuse to allow my eyes to view things that are not pleasing to God. I do have power over lust; lust does not have power over me. I do have power over my imagination and my thoughts. I refuse to entertain wrong thinking in Jesus' name.*

Power Over Fear

I am a new creation. Lust has passed away and does not have power over my life. I am a new creation and greed no longer has power over my life. I am a new creation and fear no longer has any power over my life. The person that fear had control over has been crucified with

Christ and is dead and gone. It is no longer I, the old man who lives, but Christ lives in me.

Power Over Porn

I have power over masturbation and pornography. I have power over lustful magazines, and I do not give place to the devil by viewing them. I have power over viewing porn on the Internet, and I will not view those things because they destroy my self-control over evil things. I am dead to pornography and I am completely free in Jesus' name.

Power Over Addictions

Lust and the spirit of greed are broken off of my life. I spend time every day in prayer and meditation of God's Word. I have the nature of God within me, and I have the life of God within me. Adultery, fornication, and wrong desires no longer control my life. They are broken off of me and I walk in the purity of God. I am clean through the Word of God that abides in me. I am delivered from the authority of darkness, and I am translated into the Kingdom of His dear Son. I am out of Satan's control. He no longer has any control over me and over my mind in Jesus' name.

Power Over Pride

Pride no longer controls my life because I yield my life to my Father to do those things that please Him. I am not my own, I belong to God to do His will and to be what His Word says I am. I yield my mind and my eyes to Him. I take authority over what I hear with my ears.

I refuse to allow lust, greed, or fear to become seeds in my hearing. I commit my will to God's will.

Power to Love

I love my wife (or husband), and I prefer him/her before myself. I will not use him/her to please myself. When I engage in making love, I will keep my mind and thoughts only upon him/her and no one else. I walk in the light of Your Word, Lord, and I have fellowship with You. Your blood, Lord Jesus, cleanses me from all sin and iniquity.

Power Over Generational Curses

I command every generational addiction to be broken off of my life because I am a new creation. I command every generational addiction to be broken off of my seed and my seed's seed. I take authority over unclean spirits and command them to be broken off of my life and off of my seed and my seed's seed. I command iniquity to be broken off of my life and mind in Jesus' name.

Power to Walk in the Light

Now I am free and I am walking in the light of God's Word. I will fulfill the destiny that my Father has planned for me. I will walk in love and forgive others without them asking me to forgive them. I confess that I love them with the love of God that is in my heart from being born of God. I am born of God, and I am a new creation in Christ Jesus.

13

YOUR IDENTITY IN CHRIST

Therefore if any man be in Christ, he is a new creature: old things are passed away; behold, all things are become new.

2 Corinthians 5:17

The day that Jesus sat down at the right hand of God, His work was complete and finished. The finished work of Christ is where our complete victory and deliverance from the power of darkness become a reality.

THE FINISHED WORK OF CHRIST IS WHERE OUR COMPLETE VICTORY AND DELIVERANCE FROM THE POWER OF DARKNESS BECOME A REALITY.

Many people try to become a good Christian instead of boldly declaring who they are now in Christ. Being in Christ is based on legal grounds called redemption! To understand your redemption is to understand that Satan no longer has legal power over you or your mind.

As Christians, we are in Christ. We are believers, and as believers we should know who we are in Him. One of the best ways to discover what you have is to read through the New Testament, primarily Paul's letters.

Paul's letters hold the keys to understanding what we have as a believer. Paul's writings are written to you, the believer. As you read, look for all the expressions such as, "in Christ," "in Him," and "in whom." You will find approximately 140 such expressions; most of them are found in the Epistles.

FAITH'S CONFESSION CREATES REALITIES IN YOUR INNER BEING – YOUR SPIRIT.

The Bible is a legal document, sealed by the blood of Jesus. However, it is your believing it and your confessing it which makes it a reality to you.

Faith's confession creates realities in your inner being – your spirit. Satan never has had dominion over the new creature in Christ.

I love the *Deane Translation* of Second Corinthians 5:17, **"...and the true Christian is not merely a man altered but a man re-made...."**

The man who is re-made is one like Christ, made after God in righteousness and true holiness. (Ephesians 4:24.)

The man who is re-made is one with the Father just like Jesus. (1 Corinthians 6:17.)

The man who is re-made is a partaker of the divine nature of God. (2 Peter 1:4.)

The man who is re-made is redeemed from the curse of the law. (Galatians 3:13.)

The man who is re-made is delivered from the power of darkness and translated into the kingdom of His dear Son. (Colossians 1:13.)

The man who is re-made is created after God and is made the righteousness of God in Christ Jesus. (2 Corinthians 5:21.)

The man who is re-made has the same life in him that is in God and in our Lord Jesus Christ. (1 John 5:11-12.)

The man who is re-made has the faith of the Son of God. (Galatians 2:20.)

The man who is re-made is healed and free from sickness. (1 Peter 2:24.)

The man who is re-made has the love of God in his spirit. (Romans 5:5.)

Make this confession: *I am a new creature in Christ Jesus. I am a new creation ... with the life of God ... the nature of God and the ability of God are within me.*

For more information on the believer's identity, see Pastor Brian's book called, *Discover Your Identity – The Person You Used to be Is Gone!*

Prayer

Father, I want to be a God-man – a champion for You in all aspects of my life. I want to be pleasing to You, to my wife, and to others I am involved with in family, friends, work, and church relationships.

I acknowledge Jesus Christ as Your Son, Father, and I thank You that because of Jesus' death, burial, and resurrection, I can live in wholeness and soundness of spirit, body, soul (which includes my mind, will, emotions, and intellect), relationships, and finances.

Jesus Christ is my Savior, Deliverer, and Healer. I declare myself free of all sexual perversion and addictions in Jesus' name.

I commit myself to renewing my mind daily with Your Word, Lord, and I submit my body to Your lordship. I am determined to be the God-man You want me to be, to fulfill the destiny and purpose You have given me, and to bring glory to You with my life. I desire to be a champion in my marriage and in every area of my life.

Thank You, Lord, for leading and guiding me by Your Spirit into total newness of life in Jesus' name. Amen.

Receive Jesus as Your Savior

Choosing to receive Jesus Christ as your Lord and Savior is the most important decision you'll ever make!

God's Word promises, **"If thou shalt confess with thy mouth the Lord Jesus, and shalt believe in thine heart that God hath raised him from the dead, thou shalt be saved. For with the heart man believeth unto righteousness; and with the mouth confession is made unto salvation"** (Romans 10:9-10). **"Whosoever shall call upon the name of the Lord shall be saved"** (v. 13).

By His grace, God has already done everything to provide salvation. Your part is simply to believe and receive.

Pray out loud, "Jesus, I confess that You are my Lord and Savior. I believe in my heart that God raised You from the dead. By faith in Your Word, I receive salvation now. Thank You for saving me!"

The very moment you commit your life to Jesus Christ, the truth of His Word instantly comes to pass in your spirit. Now that you're born again, there's a brand-new you!

Receive the Holy Spirit

As His child, your loving heavenly Father wants to give you the supernatural power you need to live this new life.

> **Every one that asketh receiveth; and he that seeketh findeth; and to him that knocketh it shall be opened ... If ye ... know how to give good gifts unto your children: how much more shall your heavenly Father give the Holy Spirit to them that ask him?**
>
> **Luke 11:10,13**

All you have to do is ask, believe, and receive!

Pray, "Father, I recognize my need for Your power to live this new life. Please fill me with Your Holy Spirit. By faith, I receive Him right now! Thank You for baptizing me. Holy Spirit, You are welcome in my life."

Congratulations! Now you're filled with God's supernatural power. Some syllables from a language you don't recognize will rise up from your heart to your mouth. (1 Corinthians 14:14.) As you speak them out loud by faith, you're releasing God's power from within and building yourself up in the spirit. (1 Corinthians 14:4.) You can do this whenever and wherever you like.

It doesn't matter whether you felt anything or not when you prayed to receive the Lord and His Spirit. If you believed in your heart that you received, then God's Word promises you did. **"Therefore I say unto you, What things soever ye desire, when ye pray, believe that ye receive them, and ye shall have them"** (Mark 11:24). God always honors His Word; believe it!

Please contact me and let me know that you've prayed to receive Jesus as your Savior or to be filled with the Holy Spirit. I would like to rejoice with you and help you understand more fully what has taken place in your life. I'll send you a free gift that will help you understand and grow in your new relationship with the Lord. Welcome to your new life!

Endnotes

Introduction

[1] C. S. Lewis. Summarized information regarding the "red lizard" from pages 98-103 of *The Great Divorce*.

Chapter 8

[2] Russell, Diana E. H. *Handbook on Sexual Abuse of Children,* Springer Publishing Co., 1988.

[3] The Commonwealth Fund. *Improving the Health of Adolescent Girls: Policy Report of the Commonwealth Fund Commission on Women's Health,* New York, NY, 1999.

[4] Randall, Melanie and Haskell, Lori. "Sexual Violence in Women's Lives: Findings from the Women's Safety Project, A Community-Based Survey," *Violence Against Women,* 1995, 1 (1): 6-31.

[5] Russell.

[6] Ibid.

[7] Ibid.

[8] W. E. Vine, Merrill F. Unger, and William White, Jr. *Vine's Complete Expository Dictionary of Old and New Testament Words* (Nashville, TN: Thomas Nelson Publishers, 1984, 1996), 686.

[9] Dake, Finis Jennings. *The Wordsearch 7 Dake Reference Library (CD-Rom),* Dake Publishing; Cross format from Wordsearch, edition (November 4, 2006).

[10] Ibid.

CHAPTER STUDY GUIDES

Chapter 1 – Every Man's Attraction

Part 1. Completion

1. To become a man of God, you have to come out of denial into honesty. The greatest temptation(s) or attraction(s) that pull you in a wrong direction is (are):

 ____

 ____

 ____

 ____

2. Can your mind be cleansed from wrong attractions and/or temptations? ____________ If so, how?

 ____

 ____

3. The carnal mind, which author Brian Bohrer refers to as "the little red lizard," will control the direction of your life until what two things take place:

 a. ____
 ____

 b. ____
 ____

4. Please quote Romans 12:2, which gives you the key to transformation:

____

____

____

____

5. Once you accept Jesus Christ as your Lord and Savior, how much authority does Satan have over you?

____

6. Please quote James 1:14 from *The Amplified Bible:*

____

____

____

____

____

Part 2. TRUE/FALSE - Please put a "T" in the blank if the statement is True, "F" if the statement is False.

_____7. Satan has power over a born-again Christian only as you yield to his thoughts.

_____8. James 1:14 says some men are tempted when they are drawn away and enticed by their own lusts.

Chapter 2 – The Enticement

Part 1. Completion

1. Pornography will work in your soul until it puts __________ in your mind.

2. In comparing pornography with a tattoo, you receive a tattoo in pain, but wear it in ___________; however, you receive pornography in pleasure, but wear it in ________.

3. The only thing that has the power to remove the tattoo of lust from your soul is the engrafted __________ of God. (See James 1:21.)

4. The largest groups of people viewing Internet porn are kids between the ages of __________ and ______________.

5. What is the only thing that can set you free and keep you free from the images of pornography?

   ____

6. Please quote John 15:3:________________________

   ____

   ____

   ____

   Now, personalize this verse: __________________

   ____

____

7. According to Psalm 119:9, you can cleanse your way by:______________________________

8. Please quote Psalm 119:11:____________________

____

____

____

9. The enemy wants to take you further into deception until you lose your freedom, but God wants to give you a life of ____________and ____________.

Part 2. TRUE/FALSE – Please put a "T" in the blank if the statement is True, "F" if the statement is False.

_____ 10. You cannot flirt with lust and not be hooked.

_____ 11. Lust is a deception.

_____ 12. Admitting that you are tempted is a violation of the law of positive confession.

_____ 13. The more you view pornography, the more you become desensitized to it.

Chapter 3 – Eye-Wired Men

Part 1. Completion

1. Women are stimulated by __________ ______ ________________ and by ____________, while men are stimulated by their __________ and what they see in their ______________ world.

2. To control your life, you have to starve your __________ and your ______________.

3. Please quote Job 31:1 NLT: ____________________

   ____

   ____

   Are you willing to come into agreement with this covenant and to make a commitment to walk it out? ___________

4. When lust is engaged in the imagination, chemicals are released into the _______________ center of the brain. These chemicals – serotonin, dopamine, and endorphins – are called the "__________ __________" chemicals.

5. What is the primary difference between a God-made man and a self-made man (or a predator)?

   ____

   ____

6. Do you have a plan of action or a pre-planned strategy to kill the "red lizard" in your life so you can walk in victory? ________ If so, what is your plan or strategy?

____

____

____

____

Part 2. TRUE/FALSE – Please put a "T" in the blank if the statement is True, "F" if the statement is False.

_____7. Men are eye-driven and eye-wired.

_____8. To kill the things that are out of control in your life, you must be born again.

Chapter 4 – The Enemy Within

Part 1. Completion

1. Lust, when conceived, brings forth ________, and when sin is finished with you, it brings forth ____________. (See James 1:15.)

2. List the four Greek meanings, which author Brian Bohrer gave, for the word "lust":

   a. ____
   b. ____
   c. ____
   d. ____

3. The main gate into your soul realm is the _________ gate.

4. Lust includes words and thoughts in your mind that are not in agreement with God's _________.

5. Name the three areas of worldly lust that are given in First John 2:16:

   a. ____
   b ____
   c. ____

6. According to First John 2:17, if you do the _________ of God, you will abide with Him forever.

7. An image that is in your mind long enough will create an ____________ and form a ___________.

8. Pornography destroys marriage and it destroys your __________ as a man.

Part 2. TRUE/FALSE – Please put a "T" in the blank if the statement is True, "F" if the statement is False.

_____ 9. Both men and women can be trapped in pornography.

_____ 10. Lust includes only the area of sex.

_____ 11. Lust is the enemy within which has the power to destroy you.

_____ 12. You cannot be defeated by the enemy unless he first deceives you.

Chapter 5 – The Mind Has Procreative Power

Part 1. Completion

1. Proverbs 23:7 says, "For as he thinketh in his heart, so is he...." In other words, you will become what you think on. What are some of the things you are thinking on daily?

   ____

   ____

   ____

2. God is able to transform you into a new person by helping you, through daily input and meditation of His Word, to change the way you ____________.

3. Pornography will lead to fantasy and fantasy can lead you into the Big M: ____________________. This is true for both men and women.

4. What is the primary reason you should protect your children from porn?

   ____

   ____

   ____

5. Name three of the ways the author mentions that will cause perversion and iniquity to be planted in the mind of a person?

a. ______________________________

b. ______________________________

c. ______________________________

6. To cover sin rather than confess it produces a type of rejection and a __________-controlled personality.

7. Is there a sin you need to confess to the Lord so you can be free of the guilt and shame of it? __________

   Be honest with yourself, name it, confess it to the Lord, and write out a brief strategy of how you will remain free of it:

   Challenge(s): ______________________________

   ____

   Strategy for remaining free of it: ______________

   ____

   ____

Part 2. TRUE/FALSE – Please put a "T" in the blank if the statement is True, "F" if the statement is False.

_____8. If you do not gird up the loins of your mind, at some point you will act out your thoughts.

Chapter 6 – Mastering Your Thoughts

Part 1. Completion

1. Philippians 2:5 says your mind is to be like the mind of ________ ________.

2. Just as Jesus made His thoughts His servants, you must make your thoughts your servants. What can you do to make your thoughts servants to you rather than a master over you?

   ____

   ____

   ____

   ____

3. The battleground, where the devil will tempt you, is your __________ and your ____________.

4. Have your thoughts ever driven you to yield to a temptation that you knew was wrong? __________

   Have you overcome this area of temptation, or do you still need deliverance and freedom in this area?

   ____

   ____

5. According to several scriptural passages in the book of Proverbs, Lady Lust has the ability to lure you into sin. What is your "offensive position" against her?

____

____

____

6. Ultimately, who has power over your thoughts?

____

7. You can destroy Lady Lust with __________ __________.

8. Please quote Second Corinthians 10:5: _________

____

____

____

____

Part 2. TRUE/FALSE – Please put a "T" in the blank if the statement is True, "F" if the statement is False.

_____ 9. There is little relationship between your thoughts and your lifestyle.

_____10. If your thoughts aren't your servants, they will master (control) you all of your life.

Chapter 7 – Victorious Secrets

Part 1. Completion

1. As a successful God-made man, two areas of your life that must be brought under control are:

   a. ______________________________

   b. ______________________________

2. Ephesians 5:3 AMP says, **"But ____________ (sexual vice) and ____________ [of lustful, rich, wasteful living] or ____________ must not even be named among you. . . ."**

3. "____________" is lust for money and lust to be rich.

4. The God-man's arsenal against lust includes what five things?

   a. ______________________________

   b. ______________________________

   c. ______________________________

   d. ______________________________

   e. ______________________________

5. "Accountability" means men being submitted to other men and being answerable for their ____________ and ____________.

   Is this part of your arsenal intact? ____________

   If not, what do you need to do to incorporate it into your lifestyle?

____

____

6. Another term for "mentoring" is ______________.

   Is mentoring, another part of your arsenal against lust, in place in your life? ______________

   If not, what do you need to do to include it in your lifestyle?

   ____

   ____

7. In the Greek, the word "disciple" means working through problems and finding ______________ for them.

8. Another part of your arsenal against lust is to meditate on God's ______________. Is this part of your arsenal in place? ______________ How often do you meditate on God's Word? __________

9. Imagination leads to fantasizing and fantasizing destroys marriages and intimacy in marriage.

   Have you had a challenge with imaginations that have led to fantasizing? ________________

   How can you alleviate "imaginations" and "fantasies" from your life? ____________________

   ____

10. Share a personal situation where meditating upon God's Word empowered you to overcome a temptation:

____

____

____

____

11. The fourth part of your arsenal against lust is managing your time. Do you need to make any adjustments with what you are doing with your time and/or where you are spending your time?

____

____

12. The fifth part of your arsenal against lust is integrity. The author describes "integrity" as being what four things?

    a. ____
    b. ____
    c. ____
    d. ____

13. Psalm 119:9 AMP indicates that you can be cleansed by conforming your life to __________ __________.

14. Please quote Proverbs 28:13: ________________

____

____

____

15. Write out David's prayer to God from Psalm 51:10-11, and make it your personal prayer:

____

____

____

____

____

16. The late Dr. Lester Sumrall said that the three giants that every man faces, and which he must kill, are:

    a. __________________________________
    b. __________________________________
    c. __________________________________

    Have you brought each of these giants under control in your life? ______________________

Part 2. TRUE/FALSE – Please put a "T" in the blank if the statement is True, "F" if the statement is False.

_____ 17. "Fornication" is a sexual act between people who are not married.

_____ 18. "Uncleanness" is talking about bestiality and erotic, kinky, raw things that are taking place in this world.

_____ 19. As a man, you cannot feed wrong desires and then expect to perform well in the act of marriage with your wife.

_____ 20. You will become what you think on.

_____ 21. If you don't become free of lust, it will control your life – both your present and your future.

Chapter 8 – Breaking Free

Part 1. Completion

1. Every person's goal should be to overcome the wicked one. What is your strategy for overcoming the devil in every area of temptation?

   ____

   ____

   ____

2. What does "abiding" in the Word mean to you?

   ____

   ____

3. If you believe that doing the will of God will cause you to abide forever, your response should be to ______________ yourself, just as Jesus is pure. (See 1 John 3:3.)

4. Pornography will plant iniquity in your heart and lead you on a path of ____________________.

5. The battle with sexual addiction or any other addiction begins in your ___________.

6. As a man of God, your goal should be to be free of fornication, uncleanness, and covetousness. Are you free in each of these areas?

   ____

If you are not completely free in each of these areas, what is your strategy for becoming free?

____

____

7. List the seven things cited as "open doors" to sexual addiction:

   a. ____
   b. ____
   c. ____
   d. ____
   e. ____
   f. ____
   g. ____

8. Second Corinthians 10:5 gives the key for overcoming all of the five areas of immorality – adultery, fornication, prostitution, homosexuality, and bestiality: **"Casting down** ____________________."

9. To overcome lust, you must control your ________ and your ____________.

10. Whose responsibility is it to bring every thought captive to the obedience of Christ (into obedience to God's Word)?______________________________

11. The five areas of character that need to be strengthened in every person are:

   a. ____
   b. ____
   c. ____

d. ________________________________

e. ________________________________

What specific things are you doing to strengthen these areas of character?

____

____

____

____

Part 2. TRUE/FALSE – Please put a "T" in the blank if the statement is True, "F" if the statement is False.

_____12 Sexual problems, such as lust and the "Big M," will disappear once you are married.

_____13. The Word of God has the power to expose darkness. Light always overcomes darkness.

Chapter 9 – Testimony of Allan Seals

Part 1. Completion

1. Jesus was wounded for your transgressions and bruised for your iniquities. (See Isaiah 53:5.) Explain the difference between a "transgression" and an "iniquity":

   ____

   ____

   ____

   ____

2. In the testimony of Allan Seals, he compared involvement in pornography to taking in a ______________.

   Is your life free from the input of this poison?

   ____

   If you aren't completely free, what is your plan of action for getting free?

   ____

   ____

   ____

3. Homosexuality is not a disease. It is __________. Because it is sin, you can repent, turn from it, and be free of it.

4. In his testimony, Allan Seals said, "When you were born again, you received a new nature. The old is dead, but you can keep it alive if you don't put it to death by not feeding it."

   Are there parts of your old nature that you are still feeding?

   ____

   ____

5. What are the four ways that Allan shared to feed your new nature?

   a. ____
   b. ____
   c. ____
   d. ____

6. Hebrews 9:14 says that the ____________ of Jesus Christ cleanses your conscience from dead works.

7. Write a simple prayer, asking the Lord for His forgiveness for any sins that still need to be completely removed from your life. Then in this prayer, express your acceptance of His love for you.

   ____

   ____

   ____

   ____

Part 2. TRUE/FALSE – Please put a "T" in the blank if the statement is True, "F" if the statement is False.

_____ 8. What may seem pleasurable for a moment has a hook in it if God says not to do it.

_____ 9. The closer you are to the Lord, the less you will want to sin.

_____10. When you don't receive love from a physical father, it is hard to accept love from a spiritual father.

_____11. The blood, confession of the Word, and honesty will set you free and keep you free from going back into sexual addiction.

Chapter 10 – No Temptation Is Irresistible

Part 1. Completion

1. Read First Corinthians 10:13, both from the *King James Version* of the Bible and *The Amplified Version*. Do the temptations you face come from God? ________________

   What does this verse mean to you? ____________

   ____

   ____

   ____

2. What will happen to you if you view pornography?

   ____

   ____

3. You can be king over your mind, thoughts, flesh, Lady Lust, and the red lizard as you feed upon God's __________ and meditate upon it.

   Are you spending enough time in the Word and in fellowship with the Lord? ______________

   Have you established a daily time to meet with God in the Word, in prayer, and in fellowship? Or do you need to set a regular time to do so?

   ____

   ____

Part 2. TRUE/FALSE – Please put a "T" in the blank if the statement is True, "F" if the statement is False.

_____4. There is no temptation which you cannot resist.

_____5. When you face temptation, God will sometimes provide a way of escape.

_____6. Addictions cannot rule your life unless you yield to them.

Chapter 11 – Becoming a Man of Honor

Part 1. Completion

1. The author says there is only one thing that is worse than dying and that is living without __________.

2. Please name the four keys to becoming a man of honor. You must honor:

   a. ____
   b. ____
   c. ____
   d. ____

3. The Holy Spirit is to be your mentor. He will lead you into a life of _____________.

4. As a man of honor, you must become a _________ of money rather than a lover of money.

5. Man is to honor God by honoring his __________.

6. Please quote James 4:7: ______________________

   ____

   ____

7. Please quote Hebrews 13:17: __________________

   ____

   ____

   ____

____

____

8. Marriage, as designed by God, is to reflect His glory. Does your marriage reflect God's glory?

   ____

   How can you improve in this area? __________

   ____

   ____

9. Scripture says that when you marry, you are to "leave" father and mother and "cleave" to your wife. Define the following two words in your own words:

   "Leave" - ______________________________

   ____

   "Cleave" - ______________________________

   ____

Part 2. TRUE/FALSE – Please put a "T" in the blank if the statement is True, "F" if the statement is False.

_____10. A man of honor will put God first, and he will support his family.

_____11. A man of honor will walk in the wisdom of God, and the wealth of God will follow.

_____12. A man of honor is a man of submission.

_____13. A man who is under authority will have authority.

_____14. If you honor your wife, God will honor you.

_____15. If you do not honor your wife, your prayers will be hindered.

Chapter 12 – Walking in the Spirit

Part 1. Completion

1. According to Galatians 5:16, how can you keep yourself from fulfilling the lust of the flesh?

   ____

2. The Holy Spirit, God's agent who lives in your spirit, is the One who empowers you to walk in ____________.

3. To walk victoriously over the flesh, you have to stay filled with the __________ ____________.

4. Two of the things the author says to do to walk in the Spirit are:

   a. ____________________________________
   b. ____________________________________

5. Romans 6:16 says, **"To whom ye yield yourselves servants to obey, his servants ye are to whom ye obey. . . ."** Whose servant are you?

   ____

6. How do you sow to your spirit?

   ____

   ____

   How do you sow to your flesh?

   ____

7. According to Galatians 6:8, what kind of a harvest will you reap if you sow to your flesh?

   ____

   If you sow to the Spirit?

   ____

8. You can change your actions by feeding and meditating upon God's __________.

9. Your mind will be renewed as you feed and meditate upon God's __________.

10. According to Ephesians 5:18, to walk in freedom over the lust of the flesh, you must be filled with the __________.

11. Please quote Ephesians 5:19 that tells you how to be filled with the Spirit:

    ____

    ____

    ____

    How often should you do this? ______________

Part 2. TRUE/FALSE – Please put a "T" in the blank if the statement is True, "F" if the statement is False.

_____12. You will become a servant to the thoughts you allow to live in your mind.

Chapter 13 – Your Identity in Christ

Part 1. Completion

1. Being "in Christ" is based upon ______________. When you are born again, you are redeemed, which means you move into the status of "in Christ."

2. The Bible is a legal document, sealed by the __________ of Jesus.

3. What two things will make the Bible a reality to you?

   a. ____________________________________

   b. ____________________________________

Key to Chapter Study Guides

Chapter 1 – Every Man's Attraction

1. Personal Response
2. Yes, by renewing your mind with the Word of God.
3. a. You are born again of the Spirit of God.
   b. You renew your mind with the Word of God.
4. "And be not conformed to this world: but be ye transformed by the renewing of your mind, that ye may prove what is that good, and acceptable, and perfect, will of God."
5. None! The only power Satan has over you is what you give him by yielding to his thoughts.
6. "But every person is tempted when he is drawn away, enticed and baited by his own evil desire (lust, passions)."
7. T
8. T

Chapter 2 – The Enticement

1. images
2. pleasure/pain
3. Word
4. twelve/seventeen
5. The power of the engrafted Word of God.
6. "Now ye are clean through the word which I have spoken unto you." Example of personalizing this verse: *Now I am clean through the Word which God has spoken to me in the Bible.*
7. Taking heed to [or obeying] the Word of God.
8. "Thy word have I hid in mine heart, that I might not sin against thee."

9. honor/power
10. T
11. T
12. F
13. T

Chapter 3 – Eye-Wired Men

1. words of affection/touch; eyes/imaginary
2. eyes/thoughts
3. "I made a covenant with my eyes not to look with lust at a young woman."
   Personal Response
4. pleasure/"feel good"
5. A self-made man (or a predator) yields his thoughts and imagination to produce images that over a period of time cause an action. A God-made man fills his mind and heart with the Word of God daily through reading and meditating upon it, and it changes him to become more like Jesus in both his words and actions.
6. Personal Response
   Personal Plan or Strategy
7. T
8. T

Chapter 4 – The Enemy Within

1. sin/death
2. a) Excitement of the mind; b) Longing for what is forbidden; c) Passion and inordinate affection; and d) Coveting or setting your heart on something.
3. eye
4. Word
5. a) Lust of the flesh; b) Lust of the eyes; and c) Pride of life.

6. will
7. action/lifestyle
8. honor
9. T
10. F
11. T
12. T

Chapter 5 — The Mind Has Procreative Power

1. Personal Response
2. think
3. masturbation
4. A seed of perversion is planted within them through watching pornography.
5. a) Sexual abuse as a child; b) Exposed to porn as a child; and c) Yielding to twisted thinking while watching porn.
6. guilt
7. Personal Response for all three parts of this question.
8. T

Chapter 6 – Mastering Your Thoughts

1. Christ Jesus
2. Personal Response
3. mind/thoughts
4. Personal Response
5. Personal Response
6. <u>You</u> have power over your own thoughts.
7. God's Word
8. "Casting down imaginations, and every high thing that exalteth itself against the knowledge of God,

and bringing into captivity every thought to the obedience of Christ."

9. F

10. T

Chapter 7 – Victorious Secrets

1. a) Love for money; and b) Sexual desires

2. immorality/impurity/greediness

3. Covetousness

4. a) Accountability; b) Mentoring; c) Meditating in God's Word; d) Managing your time; and e) Integrity

5. time/actions

   Personal Response

6. discipleship

   Personal Response

7. solutions

8. Word/Personal Response

9. Personal Response

10. Personal Response

11. Personal Response

12. a) truthful; b) honest; c) up-front; and d) faithful

13. God's Word

14. "He that covereth his sins shall not prosper: but whoso confesseth and forsaketh them shall have mercy."

15. "Create in me a clean heart, O God; and renew a right spirit within me. Cast me not away from thy presence; and take not thy holy spirit from me."

16. a) Lust for sex; b) Lust for money; and c) Lust for power

    Personal Response

17. T

18. T
19. T
20. T
21. T

Chapter 8 – Breaking Free

1. Personal Response
2. Personal Response
3. purify
4. destruction
5. mind
6. Personal Response
7. a) rejection of the father; b) molestation or incest; c) pornography; d) fantasizing; e) masturbation; f) calling 900 numbers; and g) immoral relationships
8. imaginations
9. eyes/thoughts
10. It is your own responsibility
11. a) loyalty; b) faithfulness; c) honesty; d) dependability; and e) commitment

    Personal Response
12. F
13. T

Chapter 9 – Testimony of Allan Seals

1. Allan Seals defines "transgression" as sin, a one- or two-time thing; "iniquity" as a bruise, which is a habitual thing.
2. poison

    Personal Response
3. sin
4. Personal Response

5. a) read the Word daily; b) go to church regularly; c) seek the Lord; and d) pray

6. blood

7. Personal Response

8. T

9. T

10. T

11. T

Chapter 10 – No Temptation Is Irresistible

1. No/Personal Response

2. Lust will rise up and control you.

3. Word/Personal Response

4. T

5. F – He will <u>always</u> provide a way of escape.

6. T

Chapter 11 – Becoming a Man of Honor

1. honor

2. a) the Holy Spirit; b) the Lord with your substance and the firstfruits of all your increase; c) those who are over you in the Lord; and d) your wife

3. purity

4. master

5. wife

6. "Submit yourselves therefore to God. Resist the devil, and he will flee from you."

7. "Obey them that have rule over you, and submit yourselves: for they watch for your souls, as they that must give account, that they may do it with joy, and not with grief: for that is unprofitable for you."

8. Personal Response

9. Personal Response
10. T
11. T
12. T
13. T
14. T
15. T

Chapter 12 – Walking in the Spirit

1. walk in the Spirit
2. freedom
3. Holy Spirit
4. a) pray in the Spirit; and b) sit under the teaching of the Word of God
5. Personal Response
6. Personal Response
7. a harvest of corruption/life everlasting
8. Word
9. Word
10. Spirit
11. By "speaking to yourselves in psalms and hymns and spiritual songs, singing and making melody in your heart to the Lord."

    Personal Response
12. T

Chapter 13 – Your Identity in Christ

1. redemption
2. blood
3. a) believing it; and b) confessing it

Resources for Men

Pure Life Ministries
14 School Street
Dry Ridge, KY 41035
888.PURELIFE
www.purelifeministries.org

New Life Ministries
P. O. Box 1018
Laguna Beach, CA 92652
1-800-NEW-LIFE (639-5433)
www.newlife.com

XXXchurch.com
Fireproof Ministries
P. O. Box 150169
Grand Rapids, MI 49515
616-588-5988
www.xxxchurch.com

Sexual Recovery Institute
822 S. Robertson Blvd.
Los Angeles, CA 90035
310-360-0130
www.sexualrecovery.com

Other Books by Brian Bohrer

Winning on the Inside –
The Road to Recovery

A spiritual journey to freedom over bitterness and unforgiveness. The author introduces you to the road that causes you to win over the things that cause most people pain. You will discover dynamic scriptural insight on topics as Overcoming the Pain of the Past, Overcoming Unforgiveness, Releasing Bitterness, How to Recover and move on with your life, Your New Identity, plus seven steps to winning on the inside.

Word Therapy –
Discover the Creative Power of Your Words

Applying God's Word by meditating and speaking His Word. Medical professionals are finding out that the thoughts of the mind and the words of the mouth are connected to many diseases in the body. God's Word tells us that positive thoughts and positive words have a healing effect upon the body. You can change your life by changing your words!

Making Peace with Your Past –
31 Days to Freedom

This is a 31-day devotional that promotes freedom. Each page contains a declaration, an affirmation, and a powerful Scripture verse. As you meditate daily on the Word of God concerning forgiveness, your life will begin to experience the peace of God that forgiveness brings.

Discover Your Identity –
The Person You Used to be Is Gone!

You will gain access into the secrets of being a new creation, secrets that were "hidden from ages and generations," but that are now revealed to us IN CHRIST.

ThinkOneCan –
Take control of your life by taking control of your attitude

"Can't" is not in the Bible. "Can" is the language of the Bible. Your attitude is a gift from God to empower your life and to attract the right people into your life. You will discover the tools to empower your life and the gift to empower others.

www.pastorbrian.org

Audio Teachings by Brian Bohrer

Lady Lust – Special teaching at Rhema Bible Church for the Call to Arms Men's Conference. Learn to avoid the bait called lust and discover four keys to being a man of honor.

Men's Locker Room Talk – A 3 CD series. Five ways to overcome lust. Breaking free from sexual sin. Sexual Addictions.

Controlling Thoughts – A 6 CD set about finances, renewing your mind, how temptation comes, and learning to have a calm, undisturbed mind.

Walking Free from Anxiety – In this 3 CD series you will learn the main keys to overcoming the influence of anxiety.

The Master's Mind – An 8 CD series on breaking free from the power of fear, guilt, condemnation, anxiety, lust, and greed.

Wisdom and Money – A 4 CD series taught in a workshop setting. Learn how to become debt-free in five to seven years and to gain wealth-building principles.

Standing before KINGS! – A 6 CD series on the 12 principles for living life at the highest level. Ideal for businessmen and women, leaders, people like you who want to achieve goals and gain success.

Lord of the Rings – 4 CD series. Discover the mysteries that make your marriage strong. Two becoming one. Strengthening your marriage. Marriage designed by God. Submitted hearts.

Marriage Designed by God – A 3 CD series. Whatever the status of your marriage today, applying these principles can produce an enhanced, successful, and satisfying relationship.

Keeping Your Marriage *Hotter Than a Pepper Sprout* – 2 CDs. A night with Pastors Brian and Kimberly Bohrer discussing marriage.

www.pastorbrian.org

For more information or to order products please contact:

Brian Bohrer Ministries
P. O. Box 1577
Washington, MO 63090 U.S.A.
Phone: 636.239.5944

www.pastorbrian.org

About the Author

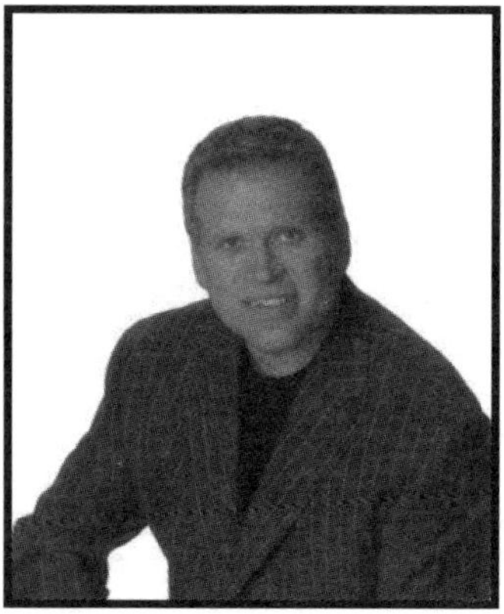

Pastor Brian Bohrer is a spiritual motivator and Bible teacher. Best known for his ability to share simple truths, seasoned with humor, Brian brings his listeners to a fresh understanding of the Word of God. Brian centers his teaching around faith and knowing who we are in Christ.

Published by 24/7 Faith Publications